DATE DUE

DEC 2 7 2005			
MAR 2 1 2006			
APR 0 6 2006			

DEMCO 128-5046

COMING TO TERM

ALSO BY JON COHEN

Shots in the Dark: The Wayward Search for an AIDS Vaccine

COMING TO TERM

Uncovering the Truth About Miscarriage

Jon Cohen

HOUGHTON MIFFLIN COMPANY
Boston   New York
2005

For information about permission to reproduce selections from this book,
write to Permissions, Houghton Mifflin Company, 215 Park Avenue South,
New York, New York 10003.

Visit our Web site: www.houghtonmifflinbooks.com.

Library of Congress Cataloging-in-Publication Data
Cohen, Jon, date.
Coming to term : uncovering the truth about miscarriage / Jon Cohen.
p. cm.
Includes index.
ISBN 0-618-27724-2
1. Miscarriage—Popular works. I. Title.
RG648.C54 2005
618.3'92—dc22 2004057676

Printed in the United States of America

Book design by Lisa Diercks
Typeset in Quadraat

QUM 10 9 8 7 6 5 4 3 2 1

For Ryan and Aidan

CONTENTS

FOREWORD

"I FEEL AS IF I'VE CROSSED A DESERT AND THEN WAS GIVEN only a sip of water," explained one of my patients, who spontaneously lost her first pregnancy following eleven years of infertility treatment. More often, patients keep their emotions to themselves rather than state them so eloquently. Yet the feeling is surely universal among those who have experienced pregnancy loss. The phenomenon is not uncommon. Miscarriage occurs in 15 percent of clinically recognized pregnancies, and 3 to 4 percent of reproductive-age couples have recurrent losses. Despite these statistics, caring physicians can recount a trove of stories recited by surprised and upset patients. Yet few couples realize how many others are going through the same grief, longing, and bewilderment. Their sense of isolation makes the situation worse.

Jon Cohen, himself a parent of multiple miscarriages, is a master at describing the real-life emotional trauma inflicted by pregnancy loss. He details the initial surprise that accompanies a first loss and follows its evolution through the diagnostic dilemmas and therapeutic indecisions, to desperation, and finally acceptance. As a contributing correspondent for *Science*, he has chronicled subjects ranging from vaccines to the HIV/AIDS epidemic. He has written on the medical cost of poverty, thus showing both scientific as well as sociological prowess. His previous book, *Shots in the Dark*, was awarded the Science and Society Award of the National Association of Science Writers. Thus, it is not surprising that *Coming to Term* is well researched, lucidly presented, and generously but not ponderously referenced. Couples can rely on the accuracy of the information. This book will benefit all couples who are infertile, or who have had a miscarriage. It may be especially valuable to those trying to decide upon therapy after multiple miscarriages.

Coming to Term is divided into three parts, appropriately titled "Mother Nature," "Mysteries," and "Hope." In "Mother Nature," Cohen describes the reproductive system and its complexities in an elementary but non-condescending manner, clearly illustrating Mother Nature's most complex but perfectly designed system. Once he brings the process of normal reproduction to life for the reader, Cohen provides the information necessary for understanding the next section, "Mysteries." There he highlights the difficulties of studying reproductive disorders. Once again, Cohen interweaves his own experiences with those of investigators and their trials. He reminds us of difficulties that arose throughout history and have led to the predicament that physicians face when treating couples experiencing miscarriages.

In "Hope," Cohen describes couples facing the decision of whether to attempt untested therapy. At least half of all miscarriages cannot be prevented by empirical, hormonal, or immunological therapy. And this is probably for the better. Researchers have found that 50 percent of miscarriages are chromosomally abnormal—some studies suggest that the rate may even be as high as 70 percent—and if those pregnancies continued to term, they would result in children who died shortly after birth or who survived with severe mental and physical problems. Nonetheless, these facts are difficult for couples to accept; they often hope that their pregnancy, regardless of the odds, was chromosomally normal. Because so many couples have shared their experiences with Cohen, the reader begins to understand why they would attempt therapy that is expensive, cumbersome, and probably ineffective. For example, carefully done studies have yet to show a clear benefit from therapy with intravenous immunoglobulin—indeed, some studies have shown no benefit at all—yet couples still try it in the hope that the "gold standard" of investigation that produced these results, the randomized clinical trial, was flawed and that perhaps for them the therapy will work. Couple after couple still attempts this futile course and other similar offerings. To his great credit,

Cohen does not condemn or ridicule, but describes and asks the reader to understand the desperation and hope that leads these patients to conclude that, no matter what the evidence suggests, success will uniquely come to them. I am reminded of a *Sesame Street* skit in which Bert and Ernie are discussing why Ernie has a banana in his ear. When Ernie explains that the reason is to keep alligators away from Sesame Street, Bert retorts, "But there are no alligators on Sesame Street." Ernie replies, "See, it's working." In part because it is so hard to lose a baby, many believe therapy that has been proven ineffective is better than nothing. Indeed, it is their banana.

Cohen knows his subject intimately. He has read the pertinent investigations in the published medical literature and has even pursued the investigators. Throughout the book, he describes his interviews with the clinicians who study miscarriage. He presents the person behind the doctor. Their personalities percolate through the opinions that they share, clearly illuminating how even the shallowest of evidence is bolstered by the strength of their convictions. Readers feel as if they are experiencing an "office visit" with these individuals. These encounters are interesting not only for patients, but also for investigators and other physicians who will enjoy meeting their colleagues vicariously.

It is never easy to lose a baby—not even when that baby is detectable only through biochemical means as a positive pregnancy test. Couples who experience repeated losses have their grief magnified by each loss and by the often conflicting advice of physicians. Frequently, well-meaning advice becomes menacing to couples searching for answers where no answer exists. Why have physicians and patients put up with such a plethora of unproven regimens? Why has miscarriage spawned so many dubious treatments? Why is such a thing tolerated, even by desperate patients?

The roots of this crisis can be found in a 1938 study by the British investigator Percy Malpas, who mathematically calculated the empirical risk of having a subsequent spontaneous abortion (the medical term for miscarriage) if couples experienced one, two, three, or more. The probability of having a fourth miscarriage was calculated to be over 90 percent. An American contemporary of Malpas, Nicholas Eastman, applied the equation to American women and calculated that they had a 95 percent chance of having a fourth spontaneous abortion. Because Eastman wrote a popular obstetrical textbook, his concept of "habitual abortion" became commonplace in obstetrics. Thus, decades of women were told that they were almost assured of having another miscarriage if they experienced three losses.

Not until 1961, when a McGill graduate student, Dorothy Warburton, actually asked women about their obstetrical history, was this erroneous concept rebuffed. Indeed, Warburton found that, in a subset of women with at least one live birth, women experiencing miscarriages had only a 30 percent chance of recurrence, without much of an increase after even four losses. Others showed that loss rates increased only marginally (perhaps 35 to 40 percent) if they had never had a live birth.

But twenty-six years of erroneous thought led to an overabundance of false concepts and ineffective therapy. If the chance of a loss was believed to be greater than 90 percent and a hypothesized therapy resulted in a 30 percent loss (the actual rate), then physicians and patients alike logically concluded that it was the therapy that actually reduced the loss! Even bed rest worked using this thinking. Thus, women with bleeding in pregnancy were sent to bed needlessly for over a quarter of a century. More importantly, if they got up from bed to take care of a child who needed them and then lost their pregnancy, they were likely to blame themselves.

Jon Cohen describes the science, the emotion, and the personalities of scientists such as Warburton as he brings alive the experience of pregnancy loss. Colorfully written and meticulously researched, *Coming to Term* is one of the best books available on the subject. I heartily recommend it to patients and doctors alike.

—SANDRA ANN CARSON, M.D.
Professor of Obstetrics and Gynecology,
Director, Baylor Assisted Reproductive
Technology Program, Baylor College of Medicine

PART ONE

MOTHER NATURE

1

···············──────···············

NOT VIABLE

ON A BRILLIANT, WARM SAN DIEGO SATURDAY IN THE SPRING
of 1996, my wife, Shannon, had her first miscarriage.

Our baffling, heartbreaking journey into the world of what doctors
call "spontaneous abortion" began with a phone call. We were having a
lazy brunch with my parents on our front porch, pine trees shading us,
the Pacific Ocean visible in the distance. Our daughter, Erin, nearly six,
was chattering with her dolls in the pine needles. Paging my way through
the newspaper, I struggled to dodge conversation with my folks, who
were visiting for the weekend and would rather talk than read. Then the
phone rang, and Shannon excused herself to answer it.

Shannon is close to my parents, but had grown weary, as had I, of my
mother's well-meaning but insensitive probing about our reproductive
status. *Any luck?* my mother would ask, month after month, noting that a
cousin of mine recently had succeeded with in vitro fertilization. *You really shouldn't wait. You really should have started earlier. Maybe you should see a
specialist. Maybe there's something wrong with your sperm. Maybe you should do
IVF. I'll help you pay for it. You two should have another. It's a shame. For Erin's
sake. She shouldn't grow up alone. My kids always had each other to play with.
There must be something you can do.*

So it was with great delight that a week earlier, we had Erin phone my
mother and tell her that Shannon, then thirty-seven, was pregnant. She
was only four weeks along, too early to see anything with an ultrasound
scan, but a blood test already had confirmed the positive urine test we had

---

3

done at home. We even had a due date. My mother squealed, really squealed, with joy. She advised us not to tell anyone else until the baby was three months along, but at every opportunity she exclaimed, "Finally!"

A few days after sharing the news, we drove to Los Angeles for Passover dinner at my aunt and uncle's house. Erin had already leaked the news to her cousins, and because Shannon's pregnancy with Erin had gone so smoothly, we ignored my mother's warning, celebrating our good fortune with all fifty of my relatives. Shannon also confided to my uncle, a doctor, that she had been spotting blood, but that her obstetrician had said it was common and usually means nothing. My uncle agreed. "Everything is probably going to be fine," he said.

Shannon's spotting continued, and we read everything we could find to help us understand first-trimester bleeding, which doctors often refer to by the frightening phrase "threatened abortion." Sometimes, when the embryo implants itself in the uterus it causes bright red bleeding for a few days. But this blood was brown and had continued staining Shannon's underwear for several days. Sometimes, bleeding occurs after intercourse because hormonal changes make a pregnant woman's cervix more exposed and delicate. Some women spot throughout their pregnancies for no known reason and without any harm to the child or the mother. Depending on whom you believe, 15 percent or 25 percent or 35 percent of women spot during their pregnancies and 25 percent or 35 percent or 50 percent of these women miscarry.

Obstetricians sometimes prescribe bed rest to prevent miscarriages, but most often they do nothing. In part, the reluctance to intervene comes from the diethylstilbestrol fiasco that surfaced in the 1970s. More commonly known as DES, this synthetic form of the hormone estrogen was widely used as a miscarriage treatment in the 1940s and 1950s. Reports began to surface in the 1950s that questioned whether DES might actually *increase* miscarriage rates, but the drug remained popular into the 1960s. In 1971, following a report that linked DES to a rare vaginal cancer in female offspring of mothers who took the drug, a bulletin from the U.S. Food and Drug Administration urged doctors to stop prescribing DES to pregnant women. Subsequent studies have found that DES caused infertility in exposed female children, genital abnormalities (of uncertain consequence) in both males and females, and may also have increased breast cancer in treated mothers. Recently, concerns have surfaced about the health of DES grandchildren.

The day we returned from Los Angeles, Shannon saw her obstetrician, who took a blood test. A six-week-old embryo should secrete increasing levels of the hormone human chorionic gonadotropin, or hCG. Home pregnancy tests turn positive when a woman's urine contains a high enough concentration of hCG. The hCG keeps a pregnancy viable by telling the body to keep producing two other hormones, progesterone and estrogen, which help prepare the wall of the uterus for implantation and prevent menstruation. The doctor told Shannon that if the embryo was healthy, hCG levels should double every two to three days.

The phone call that Saturday morning was the doctor. "I'm really sorry to tell you this, but your numbers have plateaued," the doctor told Shannon. "It's not viable. You're going to miscarry within twenty-four hours."

An ashen Shannon returned to the porch, and pulled me aside. She whispered through suppressed tears, "Ask your parents to leave." Shannon then went inside and fell on the sofa, forming a ball.

That afternoon, the intense cramps of labor walloped Shannon. By evening came the heavy, seemingly endless flow of blood that marks a first-trimester miscarriage.

Human beings are notoriously inefficient baby makers. A woman who is trying to become pregnant will succeed, on average, one out of every four menstrual cycles. According to a landmark study published in 1988, 31 percent of pregnancies end in miscarriage. So for each menstrual cycle, a sexually active woman not using birth control has less than a 10 percent chance of carrying to term. It is a wonder that we have an overpopulation problem.

Shannon and I had never thought much about fertility. We quit using birth control when Shannon was thirty-one (I'm five months younger), and she became pregnant in her first cycle. I announced our good news at my office, stupidly joking about how all I had to do was look at Shannon and she became pregnant. A woman I worked with excused herself. Later, she told me that she and her husband were having fertility problems. I learned fertility lesson number 1: your good news is not necessarily good news to others.

Shannon's first pregnancy progressed precisely as described in the stack of new books cluttering our coffee table. We marveled at each ultrasound scan, thrilling at the window into the womb and each discernible human feature of our creation. When the doctor put a microphone on Shannon's belly, we delighted to the sound of our baby's resonant heartbeat. At the baby store we bought not just a crib but, in a joyous moment that underscored how certain we were that everything would be fine, a beach chair for a one-year-old.

Everything *was* fine. Erin was born in Washington, D.C, at Columbia Hospital for Women, with ten toes, ten fingers, and no complications whatsoever. When we wanted another child, we figured, we would stop using birth control again.

We didn't want another child right away. We both had demanding careers, and we also wanted to return to our roots in California before adding to our family. And four or five years between kids seemed like the right spread, a chance for each child to enjoy our full attention.

In 1994, back in California, we rented a house with an extra bedroom and abandoned birth control again. A few months went by, but no pregnancy. The ob-gyn said not to worry: Given that Shannon was five years older, the odds of becoming pregnant in a single menstrual cycle had dropped from 25 percent to 10 percent. In a year's time, then, she should be pregnant.

But after a year, we began to suspect that something was wrong. Maybe it was me. I take a steroid, from time to time, to treat ulcerative colitis. Or maybe it was Shannon. She takes strong drugs for her migraines. Or Shannon's eggs. Or my sperm. Maybe we should see a fertility specialist. Maybe we should listen to my mother and try in vitro fertilization. Weighing these possibilities wore us down. Each of us felt guilty for secretly hoping that the other person's body had caused the problem. We worried that seeing a specialist would open a floodgate of expensive, painful, and often futile interventions. Yet as the months passed, I found myself lobbying for that option.

All that friction disappeared of course in the spring of 1996. Relief washed over us when Shannon tested positive. But the miscarriage that followed mocked us, illustrating how naïve and overconfident we had been about our fecundity.

Six months later, more frustrated still, Shannon agreed to see a specialist praised by a friend. At our first meeting, this likable doctor expressed dismay about what she saw as our casual approach to the pregnancy dance. "You're subfertile," she said. A woman's "fertility window" begins to shrink dramatically at thirty-five, she explained. We thought our odds would plummet after we turned forty, not thirty-five. The "subfertile" label chagrined us. I, in particular, wanted to read the scientific evidence behind the doctor's claims, which seemed to annoy her.

At the specialist's suggestion, Shannon started taking Clomid (clomiphene citrate), a fertility drug that stimulates an egg to mature and move to the surface of an ovary, the process known as ovulation. And on the doctor's advice, I had my sperm checked. Normal count, the lab said, but their swimming skills, daintily referred to as "motility," did not impress. After a few cycles on Clomid with no success, we upped the ante with intrauterine insemination.

On the carefully chosen day based on Shannon's ovulatory cycle, she drove Erin to school in the morning, providing me with a few minutes to deposit my seed into a sterile container before our doctor's appointment. But shortly after Shannon left, a magazine editor phoned me with deadline questions about one of my stories. When Shannon returned, the container sat empty. She was livid. "I can't believe this," she said. "I have to put my body through torture, and you can't even do the one thing you have to do. You'll do it on the way."

"I can't do that," I said.

"Get in the car," she fumed.

So as we drove along the freeway, I tried to do my thing, but, well, it's not easy when your wife is giggling at you and you're cruising down the interstate, a pea coat over your lap, in clear sight of other morning commuters sipping their coffee. As we exited the freeway fifteen minutes later, I still hadn't made much progress.

"Damn it, do it!" barked Shannon. Somehow, I did, and just as I did, I noticed a guy riding a bike staring at me.

We dropped off the container at the clinic and went out for breakfast while the lab prepared my sperm for the procedure. When we returned,

Shannon changed into a flimsy hospital gown and lay down on the examining room table. The doctors drew my sperm into a syringe and coupled it to a catheter. A team of nurses and I watched as a doctor wiggled the catheter up to Shannon's cervix and pushed the syringe plunger, sending my sperm on the journey to find one of her eggs. This isn't making love, I thought. It's making babies. The insemination failed. I was not surprised.

We tried intrauterine insemination again at the peak of Shannon's next cycle, which fell on Christmas Eve. There was holiday magic in the air. Wouldn't it be wild? Again, no luck.

The side effects of Clomid limit the number of cycles during which a woman can safely take the drug. By spring, Shannon had reached her sixth and final cycle on the ovary stimulant. Rather than try intrauterine insemination one more time, we opted for the natural approach—well, seminatural, given the Clomid—and, lo and behold, her period was late. But we did not rush to buy a $15 home pregnancy kit. Buying the kit at first suspicion, we had learned, needlessly unleashes demons. A late period has an ambiguity to it that a pee stick does not. Too many times we succumbed to the delusional drama of the pee stick, watching the second hand on the watch in frantic hopes that the test would turn positive. Too many times had we felt completely deflated both by the result and by our foolish willingness to, once again, embrace odds-defying optimism. Too many times we ended up feeling like Lotto players holding a losing ticket, cursing ourselves for having dumped money on a dream.

Our resolve gave way five days later, while vacationing in Mexico. We finally found a urine test in a dust-covered box in a little-trafficked pharmacy. We bought it anyway, and anxiously waited for Shannon's pee to highlight the enthralling "plus" symbol on the blank white stick. The stick soon showed a minus sign, but, in our delusion, we convinced ourselves that it was really a minus sign with faint traces of the plus sign poking out—if, that is, you held it in just the right light.

Were we winners or losers? On the plane home, Shannon started to spot. Her period soon followed. Her doctor later concluded that she had had her second miscarriage.

· · ·

Several months passed, and fertility and miscarriage faded into the background—at least I thought it had. One evening, Shannon asked me, her eyes wet, mascara streaking down her cheek, whether I knew what day it was. Had I missed our anniversary? "Our baby would have been due today," she said, referring to the first miscarriage. I held her as she cried and then wailed, with the particular grief that accompanies the death of someone you love.

I suffered no lasting depression about that miscarriage. In my Cro-Magnon way, I puzzled that she grieved so over a pregnancy that had lasted a few weeks. Men and women do—must—have different reactions to miscarriage, which adds yet another twist to an emotional rope that already has many knots in it. I know more intimately than anyone else what miscarriage meant to Shannon. But from another vantage, any woman who has miscarried has a more precise understanding of Shannon's sense of loss. A woman lives through a miscarriage. A man, no matter how devoted, only observes it. So Shannon's reaction to an unborn baby's birthday, a symbol that had little meaning to me at first, taught me something about what miscarriage means to a woman.

Miscarriage for Shannon did not approach the most feared tragedy that any parent can imagine: the loss of a child who actually breathes air, snuggles into your neck, and looks into your eyes. But for me, the miscarried embryo was an embryo. For Shannon, it was a son or a daughter, who, had fate been more kind, would at that moment have fed from her breast for the first time. It was that mercilessly real, and, though the pain eventually did recede, I am certain that for her it will never entirely disappear.

In the fall of 1997, Shannon and I drove to Los Angeles for a concert by Jackson Browne, whose music served as the soundtrack for our courtship when we met in 1980. The next morning, I would leave on a three-week trip to Congo, which was in the midst of a civil war. Our fears, mixed with romance, created a mystical, fated mood.

I returned from Congo unharmed, and Shannon told me she was late. Had we made a baby on a most perfect night? Was it simply a matter of all the forces in the universe aligning themselves? I do not believe in any such hooey, but for more than a moment I did. Shannon waited until my birthday to take a pee test, and this one came out strongly positive. "Happy birthday!" she announced, waving the stick in the air.

Shannon took her positive pregnancy stick to the doctor. "We love when this happens," the nurse told Shannon before taking a confirmatory sample of urine. After handing the nurse her sample, Shannon had a consultation with her doctor, which the nurse interrupted. "I'm afraid it's negative," she said.

The doctor added another phrase to our ever growing fertility playbook. "You had a chemical miscarriage," said the obstetrician, explaining that the advent of biochemically triggered pee sticks has allowed many women to see pregnancies that otherwise would have gone by unnoticed. The doctor suggested that given Shannon's age and her reproductive history, she had roughly a 3 percent chance of becoming pregnant and carrying to term.

With those grave odds and three miscarriages in two years, Shannon concluded that enough was enough. "Life is good," she told me. "I'm about to turn forty. We have a family. Let's just leave it at that." I still clung to hope, but agreed with her that we should quit actively trying to have something that nature, clearly, did not want to give us.

There surely are bigger tragedies in life than not being able to have a second child, and I soon accepted my lot in life, coming up with somewhat tortured rationales for why I was happy that things had worked out the way they had. If we *really, really* wanted another child, surely we would have pursued adoption, which neither of us ever gave serious thought. Although Erin was now only eight, it occurred to me that she was almost halfway done with living under our roof—which meant a return to freedom for us. Whenever I was near babies, I suddenly recalled how much work they required, and how much sleep they stole from their parents. And if we had another child, our two-bedroom, one-bath house would no longer work, requiring us to invest heavily in a remodel or a new home.

Why then did I feel elated when Shannon suggested that we see one more specialist? Because hope does not go quietly into the good night. It lies on its cot, suitcase packed and ready to join us anytime we invite it along.

Shannon's change of heart came about after she spoke with an old friend who had had success with the most renowned fertility doctor in town. "We should at least hear him out," Shannon suggested.

Entering the specialist's office, we noticed the requisite bounty of baby pictures overflowing from his bulletin board. He met with us after a forty-five-minute wait, guaranteeing us a 28 percent success rate if we went with in vitro fertilization. I told him a 28 percent guarantee of success equals a 72 percent guarantee of failure, and that our problem wasn't getting pregnant, it was carrying babies to term.

Yes, he understood that, but Shannon was forty, and IVF would buy us precious time by increasing the odds of a pregnancy per cycle—for about $10,000 a pop. Before investing that sort of money, we agreed on a set of tests to determine if either of us had any underlying reproductive problems. The first order of business was a sperm sample from me.

This clinic required that I produce the sample on location. On an appointed day, I joined a few other men in a special waiting room at the rear of the doctor's office. We avoided eye contact. When my name was called, a nurse ushered me into a media-equipped bathroom and showed me the magazines (including a tattered seventies-era Hustler), a TV-VCR, and a stack of porn videos. "Take as long as you'd like," she said. Right.

At our next consultation, the doctor said that because my sperm appeared normal he wanted to perform a hysterosalpingogram on Shannon. Neither of us had ever heard of this procedure, and the very sound of it, reasonably enough, frightened Shannon. The doctor explained that the test involved sliding a catheter into the uterine cavity, in the same way that they did for intrauterine insemination. He then would inject a dye into her uterus that would fill the fallopian tubes, allowing an X-ray to reveal whether her tubes were clear. It would cause some cramping, he said, but would not be painful.

We went downstairs for coffee while the doctor prepared a room for the procedure. Shannon had a meltdown, crying inconsolably. "I don't want to do this," she said. "We're done," I said, "that's it." When we told the doctor, he tried to convince us that we were making a mistake, and, unrelenting, he encouraged us to reschedule. "This isn't what we want to do," I explained. His office later phoned again to reschedule. Then he sent us a Christmas card with babies on it.

In June 1999, Shannon and I attended the Matanzas Creek Winery's annual Day of Wine and Lavender in Sonoma. The winery cultivates two acres of lavender, the aromatic, glorious herb that many cultures have celebrated for its healing properties. I put more faith in the healing powers of wine. Booking a cabin in the nearby hills and renting a convertible, we reveled in a kid-free, romantic weekend. Making a baby wasn't on the agenda.

Whether it was the wine, the lavender, the combination, or the phase of the moon, Shannon became pregnant that weekend. Urine tests are 99 percent accurate, but when she tested positive this time, we bought a second pee stick and did it again. A blood test at the doctor's office showed positive, too, and though it was too early to see the heartbeat on the ultrasound, the obstetrician—a twenty-something man we called "the Kid"—said he saw a "life form" on the machine. "Congratulations," he said, craning his neck around the machine to see Shannon's face. "You're pregnant."

Despite our history, we started to tell people. It was such great news that we just could not help ourselves. This time, we assured each other, we would be spared the need to untell. This time, everything would work out fine.

Two weeks later, Shannon returned for another ultrasound test. We well knew the drill now: If they found a heartbeat on this scan, there was a 95 percent chance that Shannon would carry a healthy baby to term. I was out of town on a business trip, and Shannon phoned me from the stairwell at the clinic. She was in a panic. "They couldn't find it," she wailed. "He said, 'It's not viable.'"

Please don't be true, we bargained with fate. *It can't be true. The Kid didn't know what he was doing.* This baby was just too perfect, conceived under perfect circumstances after we quit trying. Shannon was forty-one. This surely was our last chance. It had to be viable. It had to.

Shannon did not miscarry, and her breasts continued to grow. We returned to the Kid for a confirmatory ultrasound. He turned it on, and did a double take. "I don't know what this is," he said, pointing to a blob on the screen, "but you better go downstairs to the bigger machine." The fancier ultrasound revealed what looked like two embryos. But there was no heartbeat. Still, we asked him to have his superior look over the films that they saved from the scan. An elderly obstetrician phoned that afternoon and confirmed the Kid's diagnosis. They both said Shannon would need a D and C—a dilation and curettage, in which the doctor dilates the cervix and then uses a surgical spoon called a curette to scrape out the uterus.

Shannon wanted nothing to do with the D and C, and vowed to wait out the miscarriage. At twelve weeks, on Labor Day weekend of all things, she finally started to feel nauseated, had cramps, and miscarried. She was grateful.

Two months later, in December 1999, Shannon again was late. We did not bother to buy a pregnancy test. A few weeks went by, and our resolve crumbled. The pee stick quickly turned positive. We did not even tell Erin, nor did Shannon go see her doctor. After four consecutive miscarriages, we assumed that the fifth was a given. It was just a matter of time.

Miscarriage, no matter how much we had accepted it, represented a failure. A failure of my body or Shannon's or of our joint biochemistry, it didn't really matter: try as we might, we could not make an embryo that would attach to a uterine wall for nine months. That sense of failure I think explains why adoption held little attraction for us. We did not simply want another child. We wanted to beat what seemed a curse, to defy the experts, to, in short, succeed. But after four miscarriages, failure had thoroughly thrashed us, so much so that we both had a detached sense about this fifth pregnancy, a hardened stance that said, in effect, if we do not get our hopes up, failure will not be part of the equation. Call it denial. Call it pragmatism. We were determined not to board the emotional barnstormer, with all the nauseous loop-the-loops and barrel rolls, again.

But this pregnancy, unlike every preceding miscarriage, kept advancing just as Erin's had, just as the books described. Shannon's breasts became tender and started to swell. She did not spot at all. She had morning sickness. We bought two more pee sticks. Both turned positive nearly instantaneously. At the first doctor's visit, Shannon already was nine weeks along, and we intensely studied a monitor as a nurse performed an ultrasound scan. We had become skilled at reading the foggy sonogram images, but neither of us saw what we were looking for. The nurse did. "There it is," she said, pointing to the fetus's pulsating heart.

With a heartbeat and a positive pregnancy test, the clinic shuffled us to their obstetrician who handled high-risk cases. He performed his own scan. "This one's good from the get-go," he said.

On August 6, 2000, Shannon gave birth to our son, Ryan Yisrael Cohen.

Ryan's birth ended our personal battle with miscarriage, but the subject still gripped me, especially given how much nonsense we had heard. I decided to write the book that I wish had existed when miscarriage had us in its throes.

Early in my research, I uncovered a fact that astonished me: when "recurrent spontaneous aborters"—women like Shannon, veterans of three or more miscarriages in a row—become pregnant again, they will, with no treatment, carry to term nearly 70 percent of the time. Not only had no one ever mentioned this major detail to us, but the underlying biology baffled me. I studied miscarriage more intensively than I had during our entire odyssey with this medical malady. I wanted to separate the many myths that surround this most common event from the scientific studies that carefully have attempted to illuminate one of the greatest mysteries that exists about our bodies.

Investigating the causes of miscarriage drew me into the wonders of reproduction, tracking each step of the journey: from sperm and egg uniting into an embryo, to implantation, to viable fetus. Other species boast much higher success rates. Reproductive biologists, in particular the ones at the forefront of cloning, have begun to tease out more and more clues about what it takes to carry a baby to term.

Scientific studies prove that abnormal chromosomes account for half of miscarried fetuses. Research also clearly has established that eggs more frequently present sperm with abnormal chromosomes as a woman ages, which powerfully affects the increasing number of women who now attempt to have children in their late thirties and forties. I sought out both the researchers behind these studies and the couples participating in them to better understand chromosomal problems and their intersection with female aging, the single most common explanation for miscarriage today.

I became intrigued, too, by the many theories that tie miscarriages to aberrant immune responses. Still other studies implicate everything from coffee to Advil to alcohol. Where did the truth lie? And what role did hormones play, misshapen uteri, and infections?

As I delved deeper and deeper into the science of miscarriage, I was astonished that so little is known. The dearth of solid answers helps explain why so many unproven treatments have won wide acclaim—and remained popular even when evidence surfaces that they do not work. Scientists first raised questions about DES in the 1950s, two decades before its ban. Today, a wild, wild West mentality still exists in the miscarriage field, an oft-ignored branch of medicine. Consider some of the supposed "leading" clinicians who encourage recurrent spontaneous aborters to inject themselves with their male partner's white blood cells. A large, well-done study recently concluded that this experimental treatment results in *higher* miscarriage rates than among subjects receiving a placebo. Yet the treatment still is offered in some places. How could this be?

While Shannon and other women who repeatedly miscarry and seek help typically end up at fertility clinics, a dozen clinics devoted to recurrent pregnancy loss now exist around the world and provide much more appropriate care. As I spoke with the clinicians who run these clinics and read their many scientific publications, I became intrigued by their cutting-edge view of a problem that so many of their colleagues (many of whom make oodles of money with fertility clinics) ignore. I quickly saw, too, that recurrent loss plays the starring role in most miscarriage studies.

Recurrent miscarriage plays a starring role in this book, too. Women who have two, three, or, as befell one woman I met, seventeen, miscarriages offer insights for others. Although most women who miscarry will never have the experience again, as I discovered to my astonishment, recurrent miscarriage hardly represents a rare event, as researchers long have contended. As I will explain in some detail, modern miscarriage detection techniques have uncovered this statistic: 50 percent of conceptions fail, which means that at least half of all pregnancies fail, 25 percent of women who attempt to become pregnant likely will have two miscarriages, and 12.5 percent will have three. My intense focus on this group reflects both this new reality and the fact that for the scientists unraveling the mysteries of miscarriage, these women may hold answers that, if identified, may help the population at large.

Finally, I began to pay attention to the networks of people who offer emotional support for others who have suffered miscarriages, mostly through chat groups on the Internet. Some have tragic tales of unrelenting despair, while others, like us, have happy endings. Most everyone reaches a tone of honesty and clarity that death, uniquely, ushers in.

Disease binds people. Look at the coalitions that have formed around AIDS, breast cancer, and diabetes. But miscarriage, as common as it is, does not qualify as a disease. It is not even a medical condition. That orphan status, mixed with the taboo of discussing miscarriage and the many scientific unknowns, feeds the loneliness and confusion that many of us feel when we are in the throes of such a sad experience. I hope this book will encourage people to talk more openly about their own miscarriages, and that it also provides an accurate assessment of what science understands, and what, as of yet, it does not.

The book weaves together personal stories with the most authoritative scientific research that I could unearth, which I have divided into three parts. After explaining my personal history and impetus for writing the book, the first part, "Mother Nature," examines the fundamental biology of reproduction, with close attention paid to the genetics, the single most important driver of miscarriage. Part Two, "Mysteries," looks closely at several leading theories about what causes miscarriages of genetically normal embryos and fetuses, exploring in depth the various interventions that attempt to prevent them. I first look at immune causes of miscarriage and treatments, which range from the theoretical to the proven to the disproved. Hormonal problems follow, again with a critical eye cast toward the many experimental interventions now available, and leading to a sobering look at how DES, a synthetic version of estrogen, became a popular miscarriage drug. DES caused anatomical abnormalities, but many others occur naturally, and I focus on their effects and attempts to correct them. Part Three, "Hope," opens with an examination of the long list of environmental and lifestyle factors that miscarriage researchers have dragged down to the station house and put under the harsh light. I then profile three clinics, each in a different country, that specialize in miscarriage, describing what state-of-the-art care looks like, as well as a myriad of patients who have many of the problems described in earlier chapters. The book closes with a few of the most extraordinary miscarriage stories I came across.

People repeatedly have asked me why women would want to read a book about miscarriage written by a man. Well, why wouldn't they? And why wouldn't men? If my book aimed to explain how it felt physically and emotionally to miscarry, and how to handle the grief, I think a woman writer who had experienced a miscarriage inevitably would offer unique, powerful insights. But the questions that interest me most evade special claim because neither gender knows more when it comes to puzzling out how the human body works and devising strategies to help it when something malfunctions. Why do miscarriages happen? Which interventions work, which ones might, and which ones do not? Women and men alike struggle mightily to unravel these mysteries. If one or the other has an edge, I have not seen it.

I well recognize that Ryan is a gift, even a miracle, and that a happy ending eludes many couples who struggle with miscarriage. Still, for couples who have had miscarriages and still hold out hope, this book makes the case that their prospects might not be as bleak as they seem. And regardless of whether couples who badly want a child ever realize their dreams, this book ultimately concludes that we all must come to terms with our reproductive fates, which, try as humans might, we have less control of than we would like.

2

THROUGH A GLASS, CLEARLY

FROM THE START, LIFE DODGES DEATH.

At the five-month mark, a female fetus will have produced all of the eggs that she will carry during her lifetime. Then a subtraction game begins. The 7 million or so oocytes park in the two oval-shaped ovaries. For reasons that still elude scientists, shortly after the egg cells come into existence they begin to self-destruct and this suicide continues throughout a woman's reproductive years. At birth, the baby girl's ovaries will contain only 1 to 2 million eggs. By the time she reaches puberty, her ovaries will carry but 200,000 to 300,000 eggs. These eggs actually compete to reach the surface of the ovary, with a mere 400 to 500 succeeding over the span of a woman's life. Menopause arrives not at a certain age, but when the ovarian reserve falls to about 1,000 eggs.

An understanding of miscarriage hinges on these facts. And the more exacting the details that science can uncover about how an egg becomes a viable fetus, the more likely it is that clinicians will discover effective means to prevent pregnancy loss.

When an egg wins the competition and squeezes through the cellular wall that surrounds an ovary, it enters a new world. The egg first bursts out of its protective sac, the follicle, which later plays a critical role if fertilization occurs. Shrouded in a cloud of cells, this egg usually finds itself swept up by the delicate fingers on the ends of the fallopian tube nearest its ovarian home. As the fingers move the egg into the wide end of this moist funnel, the microscopic hairs that line its walls take over, slowly moving it down the four-inch path that leads to the human incubator, the uterus, more commonly known as the womb. On all but the rarest of occasions, the egg, which measures about one-tenth the width of a human hair, will not meet any gentlemen callers along this journey, the uterus will shed its lining, and a menstrual period will follow. Researchers do not know that egg's fate, but they suspect that somewhere along the way it disintegrates, the detritus lost in the eight teaspoons or so of blood that typically constitute menses.

But if a woman has intercourse no earlier than five days before and no later than one day after that egg surfaces on the ovary, a much different, and more dramatic, story can play out.

As with eggs, the overwhelming majority of sperm never come close to making a baby. When a man ejaculates into a woman's vagina, a few hundred million sperm, on average, arrive on an unwelcoming foreign beach. First, the sperm face what many textbooks refer to as the "hostile environment" of the vagina, which has a high acidity that can fry them. Sperm elude this potential killer by donning a uniform of alkaline fluid, contributed by the prostate, which buffers the acid—at least for a short while. The sperm that, by wagging their tails, move up to the cervix most often find a thick mucous plug that bars this gateway to the uterus. Midway into a menstrual cycle, though, a thinner, friendlier mucus appears that allows sperm either to pass through or to hang out for several days in acid-free safety.

Sperm that leave the cervical mucus must next navigate past the deep crypts of the cervical canal and into the uterus, which has the shape of an upside-down pear and measures a mere two inches wide and three inches long. By then, the sperm ranks have dwindled down to a few hundred thousand. Before sperm can properly fertilize an egg, they must mature. First, the uterus steps in as a *valet de chambre*, grooming select sperm with biochemicals that strip off parts of the sperm's membranes, hyperactivating them. Aimlessly racing about like kids driving bumper cars, these frenzied sperm rely on uterine contractions to make their way toward the two fallopian tubes. From the several hundred million that started out, only about 250 travel-weary sperm will ever find their way to a fallopian tube.

During its odyssey, the egg communicates with the ovary. In a poorly understood process, the egg transmits chemical signals that cause the fallopian tubes to contract, propelling the sperm toward the ultimate conjugal act. To fulfill its destiny, a mature sperm must nosedive through the cloud of cells around the egg and dock onto its zona pellucida, a transparent sphere that forms a jellylike outer membrane. In fine top-gun form, the sperm then takes aim at the zona and fires a bolus of enzymes, which it has stashed away in its nose cone. Twenty minutes later, with help from the enzymes and its whiplashing tail, the sperm will bore into the zona and enter the inner sanctum of the egg. As the sperm head fuses with the plasma membrane of the egg, it jettisons its tail and dumps its genetic cargo. The zona pellucida simultaneously transforms into a hardened shell, rebuffing all other sperm that subsequently come knocking.

While the sperm arrives with twenty-three chromosomes, the egg has forty-six, an extra copy of each one. The process known as meiosis separates the forty-six into two identical sets of twenty-three, pushing one set into a spherical trash sack called a polar body. At long last, the 23 male chromosomes find their identical female dancing partners. After a few twirls this way and that, the chromosomes will intertwine their arms and legs with the final intercourse of intercourse. A zygote is born. As if to mark this birth, the egg ejects the polar body, a small balloon filled with surplus DNA that floats away into oblivion.

Leaving aside the intractable and knotty debates about when life begins, we do know that about half of all human zygotes die before completing their journey down the fallopian tube and implanting in the uterine wall. These losses receive little attention because science has yet to devise a method that can routinely detect them, but they represent the earliest form of miscarriage. For the zygotes that survive, researchers have invented a wondrous collection of words to describe the budding human that, until the advent of fertility clinics, rarely appeared outside the halls of science.

After about one day, a healthy zygote divides into two cells, each called a blastomere, Greek for "sprout part" — we do spring to life! — and they continue to cleave into four and then eight blastomeres at about the same leisurely pace. At day three or four postconception, sixteen to thirty-two blastomeres clump into a morula, the Latin word for "mulberry." The morula floats for two or three days in the uterus, nourished by secretions from glands in the membrane that lines the uterine wall. After a few more divisions, a profound change occurs: the morula becomes a blastocyst, or "sprout bladder."

At roughly six days after fertilization, the blastocyst hatches—yes, hatches—from the egg shell, and the process of implanting into the uterine surface, or endometrium, begins. Special cells from within the blastocyst, ones with little hairs sticking from their surfaces, dock onto a flowerlike structure that buds from the endometrium so that the hairs interlock with the tiny "petals." Slightly different cells from the blastocyst then invade the endometrium, spitting out enzymes that cut through the tissue and allow the blastocyst to implant itself deeper.

In concert with the blastocyst's invasion of the endometrium, an increasingly diverse stream of biochemicals ripples this way and that to help the embryo properly embed itself. Back at the ovary, the busted follicle that once held the egg cell sends the hormone progesterone to help the uterus receive the blastocyst. A steady stream of white blood cells and immune system messengers counsel the mother's body to accept this aggressive newcomer, which behaves like a tumor, relentlessly doubling in size with an agenda of its own. Some women will spot a little from the bleeding caused by implantation.

Ten days after fertilization, the conceptus has burrowed itself completely into the womb's wall. Blood vessels from the mother begin to nestle against tendrils that grow from a primitive version of the placenta. By the two-week point—at which a woman would first notice that her period was late—the embryo floats in a protective balloon of amniotic fluid, and a placenta rich in blood vessels stands ready to feed it. A distinctive line called a "primitive streak" surfaces, marking the first transition from a clump of cells into specific body parts. The placenta also pumps out enough of the hormone human chorionic gonadotropin (hCG), which circulates only after implantation, to turn a pregnancy test positive.

Now the embryo develops familiar parts. The nervous system emerges during the third week, fashioning a tube that will in time become the spinal cord and the brain. An S-shaped organ that will become the heart begins to form and pump fluids. During the fourth week, the embryo looks like a minuscule hammerhead shark with limb buds popping out from its sides. It measures less than half an inch and weighs less than a gram. By week five, the embryo has pits for eyes and a nose. At week six, the bones begin to harden, and the tip of the nose becomes distinct, as does the lower jaw and the outlines of the fingers and toes. The woman also misses her second period. The next week the gonads form. Brain waves become detectable, and knees and elbows take shape. Week eight separates an embryo from a fetus, as all essential structures have developed.

More than 90 percent of miscarriages occur by the eighth week.

This sharp picture of the first eight weeks of life exists thanks to decades of work by legions of developmental biologists. No such cadre of researchers live and breathe miscarriage, in part because it's incredibly difficult to capture the unraveling of early life. But some investigators have made headway, and I went to great lengths to seek them out.

With each successive miscarriage, Shannon and I became increasingly frustrated with the mumbo jumbo we kept hearing from the specialists about what had happened, what we should do, and how we should view our prospects for having more children. Not only did different doctors give us wildly different explanations, but when I pressed for scientific studies that we could consult no one had anything to offer, and some had the audacity to shift into the all-wise-M.D. mode, counseling us to accept the losses and try again. We wanted facts, and one day it dawned on me that I make my living ferreting out scientific facts. Why not take the plunge myself into the scientific literature for the real story?

Because the genesis of eggs plays such a central role in miscarriage, I began with the oft-repeated "fact" that the female fetus makes 7 million eggs by the fifth month postconception. Who discovered that number and how?

Several scientific papers pointed to a study published in 1963 in the *Proceedings of the Royal Society, Biological Sciences*. Written by a sole author—an oddity in modern biology where collaboration rules—the paper by

T. G. Baker from England's University of Birmingham focused on ovaries removed from fifty-six fetuses, five newborns, and fifteen prepubertal "specimens." The utterly convincing paper documented how the number of eggs peaked at 6.8 million a mere five months after conception. By the time of birth, 4.8 million have died, and by seven years of age, only 300,000 remain.

I soon reached Terry Baker, the author, on the phone. "I had a marvelous collection of material," Baker, now a professor emeritus at the University of Bradford in Yorkshire, told me. How, I wondered, had he collected all of these "specimens"? Many came from miscarriages. "My motto throughout my career has been: Nature produces mistakes that lead us to really important discoveries." This notion would become a recurring theme as I delved deeper into the mysteries of miscarriage. Baker explained that Britain's relatively lenient abortion laws made the collections of specimens easier.

Baker's report had a dramatic impact on science's understanding of how human females make and destroy eggs, which, I would soon discover, helps explain some of the most fundamental reasons why miscarriages occur—and why they become more common as women age. And I became intrigued by how, in the world of science, abortion overlaps with miscarriage—which medicine refers to as "spontaneous abortion"—a phenomenon that extends far beyond Terry Baker's work.

In a cavernous room at the Armed Forces Institute of Pathology in Washington, D.C., rows of file cabinets hold an astonishing collection of seven hundred embryos that offer the most detailed view imaginable of how human life begins—and prematurely ends. Known as the Carnegie Collection of Embryology, the samples stretch back to 1887, and they exquisitely document each stage of development from conception through the first eight weeks of life.

Liz Lockett, a medical illustrator who helps oversee the collection, opens the first file drawer, which holds the youngest embryo. Viewing the embryo through a microscope, researchers cut each specimen into cross-sectional slices that measure but eight to ten microns thick—the size of an unfertilized human egg. They spent three to six months preparing each embryo, Lockett tells me with obvious wonder. "They literally lost not a single section," she says. The slices, sandwiched between glass slides, now sit in little wooden boxes, arranged sequentially. The first embryo occupies nine of these boxes, and, as we move down through the collection, each successively older embryo, owing to the increasing size, requires ever more wooden boxes.

Lockett opens a drawer that holds one of the embryos that led me here, a small subset of the Carnegie Collection put together by Arthur Hertig and John Rock, who from 1938 to 1954 conducted a remarkable experiment that no one would dare attempt today.

Rock, a prominent ob-gyn at both Boston's Free Hospital for Women and the Lying-In Hospital teamed up with Hertig, a younger pathologist at both institutions, on what became known as the "egg hunt." At the time, science knew next to nothing about how life actually began. "No one knew what a human embryo looked like during the first two weeks of life, nor exactly when conception took place, or where, and nothing was known about when or how the young conceptus implanted in the lining of the womb," Hertig explained to Rock's biographer.

Hertig and Rock came to the question from different angles. Hertig, who had abandoned a career investigating the relationship between insects and human diseases to study obstetric pathology, had become a specialist in the placenta and miscarriage in particular. After completing his medical degree at Harvard, he studied the relationship between formation of the placenta and miscarriage at the Carnegie Institution of Washington with the director of embryology, George Streeter. "Dr. Streeter was the only embryologist, together with his colleague Dr. Chester H. Heuser, who seemed to know or even care about the pathogenesis of spontaneous abortion," Hertig once wrote, referring to the chain of events that cause miscarriage.

Rock, a devout Catholic who later would play an instrumental role in developing the first birth control pill, ran a clinic that both taught the rhythm method and assisted infertile couples. At his instruction, patients kept charts of their intercourse.

As with most ob-gyns, Rock routinely performed hysterectomies.

What if he selected women from this group who already had given birth and had no known fertility problems, and asked them to chart their intercourse before the operation? By timing surgeries to follow a predicted ovulation, he increased the odds that the removed fallopian tubes or uterus might carry an embryo. "Both Rock and Hertig thought about the ethical implications long and hard," wrote Loretta McLaughlin in The Pill, John Rock, and the Church. According to McLaughlin, they saw it as a "necessary scientific endeavor using material that would have gone to waste but would not have been put to the use for which the Lord intended it."

Neither investigator, she noted, regarded "the conceptuses they hoped to find to be abortuses." This is wordsmithing: an "abortus" simply refers to a "conceptus" outside of the body. But in Hertig and Rock's defense, no test then existed that would reveal such an early pregnancy in the women they recruited.

During the sixteen years of their study, Hertig and Rock examined the uteri and tubes from 211 women, "recovering" 34 fertilized ova that ranged from two to seventeen days old. Of these, a staggering 13 — or 38 percent — showed evidence of abnormality. Four of the thirteen abnormal embryos had yet to implant. The study also found four normal embryos at that early stage. So a whopping 50 percent of the early embryos Hertig and Rock found had serious problems. Although they cautioned that it "is impossible to say how many of these abnormal pregnancies would have terminated in spontaneous abortions," they also thoroughly categorized problems that make it seem likely that most, "would have been merely swept away with the unsuppressed menstrual flow."

Lockett takes a box of slides that holds sliced-up pieces of one of the Hertig and Rock embryos, No. 7081, and we look at them under a microscope. The individual slices from one perspective resemble a piece of prosciutto, while from another I see a faraway shot of a Martian landscape with dried riverbeds coursing through valleys and into oceans that contain islands. With Lockett's help, I can identify the embryo and the nascent placenta in this thirteen-day-old embryo, one of the normal ones they found. Other shots show the intact embryo implanted in the uterine wall.

Hertig and Rock published dozens of papers about their collection, most all of which contain abundant photos made from these slides. I want to see miscarriage in action, and these thirteen cases offer the most up-close view science ever has captured. So I study these photos, learning to read what seems like hieroglyphics. Their accompanying text also makes plain what my eye would never, on its own, have noticed, and offers theories of causation that turn my head around.

My favorite Hertig and Rock papers offer peculiar snapshots, both of the women and their embryos. The papers sketch the obstetrical histories of the women, detail their intercourse ("coital dates") prehysterectomy, and then show several photos of each specimen both intact and in cross section. Together, the images provide something of a filmstrip of life's origins, as they move chronologically from the youngest embryos to the oldest.

No. 8630, the youngest abnormal embryo, has but five cells, and the doctors estimate that it was four days old. The woman, Mrs. P.B., had a prolapsed uterus—a hernia-like condition in which it drops into the vagina—and had suffered irregular periods for five months. She had had three children and one documented miscarriage. Hertig and Rock note the variable shapes of the five cells and the odd-looking nuclei. In contrast, healthy embryos at this stage exhibit a gorgeous symmetry.

The researchers posit that "delayed fertilization" may have caused the abnormality. As Mrs. P.B.'s records show, she had sex 84, 132, 156, and 204 hours before the operation. Based on her past menstrual cycle, they presume that she ovulated 108 hours before the operation. If the couple had sex 84 hours before operation, "the ovum would have been stale and probably not normally fertilizable," they assert.

The next abnormal specimen, No. 8450, had eight cells with similar defects. Mrs. M.B., thirty, had six children, one documented miscarriage, and one self-induced abortion. She clearly had a troubled life. "Because of a difficult socio-economic and psychological situation in her home, two psychiatrists and the obstetrical staff of another hospital advised sterilization," note Hertig and Rock. They theorize that an excessive amount of sex may have caused the formation of an abnormal embryo. "It is possible that the performance of coitus six times within twelve days may have caused some drop in the number and change in the morphology of the spermatozoa," they conclude.

The older, more developed embryos they recovered raised questions that still beguile reproduction specialists. When an ovarian follicle releases an egg, the follicle becomes a corpus luteum, a yellow mass of cells that secretes the critical hormone progesterone. Aberrations riddled the corpus lutea in most of the nine implanted but abnormal embryos that the two investigators harvested. They note in their writings the embryo-and-egg problem: it's unclear whether the corpus luteum itself had a problem or whether the abnormal embryo did not send the proper chemical signals to the growing corpus luteum. The site of implantation might also have played a role, as the healthy embryos were two times more likely to have nestled into the side of the uterus facing the woman's rear. In some specimens, normal-appearing embryos were developing abnormal-appearing placentas and, as Hertig wrote in a monograph, were "destined to die at some stage of development with consequent spontaneous abortion." White blood cells had infiltrated one perfectly normal embryo, raising the possibility that the mother's immune system might ultimately have rejected it.

In McLaughlin's Rock biography, published in 1982, she explains that she found only two news articles that referred to the Hertig and Rock work, one from 1939 and the other from 1966. "Amazingly, while the Hertig-Rock collection of fertilized eggs was regarded as one of the pinnacles of research among embryologists, the public knew next to nothing about it." Amazing, yes, but I am not in the least surprised that the miscarriage aspect of the work received scant interest outside of scientific circles. As Hertig noted, miscarriage mostly interested the public and scientists alike only when studies explored treatments. Fundamental biological insights had no obvious value, a point that riled Hertig. "In a general vein, the author deplores the vast literature on the treatment of threatened abortion which does not contain much evidence that the clinician or pathologist bothered to examine the tissue from the therapeutic failures," he wrote in *Human Trophoblast*, a monograph published in 1968, when he was sixty-four.

The lack of interest may have something to do with the challenge of studying abortuses. In the monograph, Hertig quotes a fellow pathologist as saying "it takes far longer to look at an abortus or a placenta than any other surgical specimen, even a complete set of tubes, ovaries and uterus!" And the ever blunt Hertig offers this advice: "Unless a pathologist is willing to learn, or relearn, a bit of normal human embryology, look at the specimen with tender-loving care, and think about what probably took place during the six to seven weeks of development preceding the abortion, he might better throw (or urge the clinician to throw) away the material."

During his career at Boston's Lying-In Hospital, Hertig examined one thousand miscarriages, which he reported in great detail. To him, the study of abortuses offered more than just pure scientific information. "[I]t is comforting to the patient and her obstetrician to know what the abortus shows," Hertig wrote. "Most patients believe that it is due to moving of furniture, a heavy washing or some other household chore. The well-attached, normal ovum in a normal uterus survives all manner of psychic and or traumatic shock, the legal profession to the contrary and notwithstanding."

Hertig divided the miscarriages he studied into two broad categories. "Ovular factors" refers to eggs, embryos, or placentas that have clear abnormalities, which accounted for 617 of the 1,000 miscarriages he examined. The second category, "maternal factors," covers everything from "criminal abortions" to abnormal uteri, disease, and, intriguingly, only one case of trauma.

I did not find any descriptions from Hertig and Rock that provided a reverse of the well-documented, magnificently illustrated accounts of the healthy, growing embryo rolling down the tube and implanting itself in the endometrial wall of the uterus. But Hertig, who died in 1990 and probably knew more about miscarriage than any scientist of his time, did offer a simple description of what he called the "final casting off of the conceptus." It is, he wrote, "merely a delayed menstrual period and is caused by the same factor—hormonal withdrawal of endometrial support."

That description has a particularly satisfying resonance because of the murky dividing line between a woman experiencing a delayed menstrual period and a pregnancy, especially during the days when Hertig and Rock conducted their landmark studies, when most women who had miscarriages never would have known they had conceived a child. Rather, a few months might pass between conception and confirmation of a pregnancy. First, a woman would have to see her doctor for a pregnancy test, which she logically would not do until after she missed her period. The test itself required sending a sample of urine to a laboratory, which would inject it into a female rabbit. If the urine contained high levels of hCG (human chorionic gonadotropin)—the main biochemical marker of pregnancy then and now—a large hemorrhagic mass would bulge in the rabbit's ovaries. (To see this phenomenon, the early tests required killing the rabbit, leading to the mistaken notion that if the rabbit died, the woman was pregnant. In fact, all of these rabbits died, regardless of the test's outcome.) The lab of course would then have to send its results back to the doctor, who would have to contact the patient.

Underscoring how frequently women mistook miscarriages for late periods, Hertig and Rock repeatedly noted that 10 to 15 percent of clinically recognized pregnancies ended in miscarriage. Not only did their own findings make plain how much more miscarriage actually occurred, but the advent of simpler, more rapid tests for hCG—the basis of the modern home pregnancy urine test—strongly has confirmed Hertig and Rock's observations.

The anatomist Dixon Boyd, a contemporary of Hertig and Rock, who worked at the University of Cambridge from 1951 to 1968, compiled his own collection of embryos, fetuses, and placentas from hysterectomies, stillbirths, and abortions, and the few hundred specimens illustrate the mechanics of miscarriage. Conventional wisdom once held that blood flows to the placenta from the mother as early as seventeen days after conception. But research in the late 1980s upended this notion and in the late 1990s scientists studying the Boyd Collection took it further still with solid evidence from ultrasounds, abortions, and hysterectomies that shows no significant maternal blood flows to the placenta until the twelfth week. This finding shines a high-powered light on the process of early miscarriage.

Babies and mothers do not start out as one. They are completely separate in the early going and don't merge until the embryo affixes to the uterine wall. As Boyd and others established in 1960, cells from the placenta invade the mother's arteries in her uterus during implantation and create a maternal-fetal conduit to feed the baby oxygen and carry away wastes. But as Boyd discovered, placenta cells exercise a tight grip on the spigot that controls the flow of blood from mother to baby. Specifically, the placental trophoblasts that drill into the maternal arteries immediately plug them. Blood starts to flow to the conceptus only when these trophoblast plugs loosen.

For decades, researchers believed that the unplugging occurred early in the first trimester, but in 1987 a Belgium team of scientists challenged this timing with several lines of evidence that little blood flowed to the fetus until the second trimester. Building on this finding, Cambridge's Graham Burton, working with his longtime collaborator Eric Jauniaux from University College London and colleagues, examined twelve Boyd specimens whose gestational age (based on the mother's last menstrual period) ranged between 43 and 130 days. They discovered that the embryo trophoblasts that invade the mother's arteries plug the maternal arteries until the eighth week, at which point they loosen their grip and allow blood into the materno-fetal interface, a part of the placenta called the intervillous space. The treelike chorionic villi that give the placenta its characteristic appearance bathe in this blood, exchanging material between mother and fetus. At about the twelfth week, the mother's spiral-shaped arteries begin freely spurting blood into the intervillous space.

This observation raised a profound question: What nourishes the embryo during the first weeks of life? Turning to the Boyd Collection again, Burton's team analyzed ten specimens, aged 43 to 87 days, and found evidence that glands in the uterine lining secrete nutrients into the intervillous space. Other mammals feed their embryos and fetuses with such "endometrial milk." The researchers concluded in a 2002 paper that the endometrial glands "play a more major role in early human pregnancy than previously recognized, and their malfunction could be a factor in early pregnancy loss."

In more detailed studies of intervillous circulation and miscarriage, Burton's team reported in June 2003 one of the most precise descriptions of how early losses occur. "The premature entry of maternal blood into the intervillous space at this stage of pregnancy disrupts the placental architecture and is probably the mechanical cause of most miscarriages," they wrote. So if this assertion holds, faulty plugging of spiral arteries leads to the maternal blood prematurely bathing the placenta, harming its structure and directly causing miscarriage.

A framed picture on the wall of Allen Wilcox's office shows a collage of baby photos, the type of artwork that has become standard fare at ob-gyn offices and fertility clinics everywhere. But underneath this collage, Wilcox has hung a framed cover of *Newsweek* magazine from August 15, 1988, that more accurately reflects the fruit of his labors. The photo on the cover shows an empty bassinet. "Miscarriages," reads the headline. "As Many as 1 in 3 Pregnancies Fail. Doctors Are Just Beginning to Understand Why."

Wilcox, an epidemiologist at the National Institute of Environmental Health Sciences in Research Triangle Park, North Carolina, headed a study that has yielded the most precise information on the rate of miscarriage ever collected. Between 1982 and 1985, Wilcox and his colleagues placed classified ads in a local paper, among the garage sale notices, hunting for women willing to join the Early Pregnancy Study. The ambitious study required women to collect their morning urine each day and keep it in the freezer. At the end of the week, Wilcox's team would collect the samples and distribute another week's worth of empties. The women also would have to note on a daily record card whether they had had unprotected sexual intercourse, symptoms of pregnancy, or vaginal bleeding. For their cooperation, women received $10 a week for up to six months.

Wilcox, who is an M.D. as well as a Ph.D. in epidemiology, launched the study because of an infamous cluster of miscarriages in the Love Canal section of Niagara Falls, New York. As New York State Department of Health researchers had discovered in 1978, women who lived in homes built atop a former chemical waste dump reported an alarmingly high number of miscarriages. "But the observations relied entirely on the women's own reports of miscarriages," says Wilcox. "There's a gray area here, and that led me to ask how much miscarriage really occurred."

Wilcox teamed up with a researcher at Columbia University in New York who had just developed an ultrasensitive test that could detect minute amounts of hCG. (The test is one hundred times more sensitive than over-the-counter urine kits.) For several years, Wilcox regularly shipped frozen urine samples from North Carolina to New York. In the end, the researchers analyzed a staggering 29,000 urine samples taken from 221 women. Wilcox's colleagues dubbed him the "King of Pee."

The hCG test detected 198 pregnancies, and 31 percent of these ended in a miscarriage. More revealing, most of these miscarriages had gone undetected by the women. If the study simply tallied pregnancies that women suspected and then had confirmed by a clinician, the miscarriage rate would have been only 9 percent. This statistic roughly agrees with several studies that have reported a *clinically diagnosed* miscarriage rate of about 15 percent.

The Wilcox study rewrote the book on miscarriage. Not only was the miscarriage rate more than double what most clinics recognized, but women much more frequently had two or more miscarriages than was commonly assumed. Researchers long have relied on a simple equation to calculate the risk of recurrent miscarriage in those who have no underlying problem that causes losses: If a woman has a 15 percent risk of one miscarriage, then her risk of having two miscarriages is 15 percent multiplied by 15 percent (2.25 percent), and so on. The risk that a woman will have three miscarriages, by this equation, becomes a tiny 0.3 percent.

Plugging in Wilcox's finding that 31 percent of pregnancies miscarry at implantation, the risk of two miscarriages becomes 9.6 percent, and the risk of three, 3 percent—ten times higher than the previous estimates.

But Wilcox analyzed miscarriage only *after* implantation; remember, Hertig and Rock found eight preimplantation embryos, and half exhibited serious abnormalities. Undisturbed by the doctors, such embryos may never implant, and thus escape the detection of an hCG test, leading many miscarriage researchers to assume that at least half of all conceptions fail. If even the 50 percent figure holds true, then the risk of having three losses rises to 12.5 percent, hardly a rare phenomenon.

The gap between the real and the perceived frequency of miscarriage has decreased markedly since the Wilcox team conducted their study, and it promises to continue to shrink. In 1982, when women started donating their daily urine samples for this study, home pregnancy tests had been on the market for only three years. The supersensitive ultrasound probe put inside the vagina—as opposed to the familiar wand on the belly—did not yet exist. Today, thanks to these advances, women can detect pregnancies and miscarriages that twenty years ago routinely would have escaped notice. The upshot: as more women use these new tests, miscarriage rates inevitably will appear to climb, and, eventually, clinicians and patients alike will start to view recurrent miscarriage as fairly common.

Already, many clinicians recognize that, in healthy mothers, miscarriage is as common as birth. And the ones who have examined the Wilcox results closely will recognize that it carries a terrifically upbeat message: 95 percent of the women who miscarried—including three who had two losses—conceived during the next two years. "For most women, early losses are a sign that things are working," says Wilcox. "They've made it over lots of hurdles." Driving home this point, Wilcox notes that the fourteen women in the study who failed to conceive over the same two-year period had only three detected miscarriages among them. Odd as it might seem, miscarriage, then, often represents a sign of hope.

Results from the study appeared in a 1988 issue of the *New England Journal of Medicine.* That prestigious journal also published two other articles based on Wilcox's urine collection. One 1995 paper examined the relationship between the timing of sexual intercourse and ovulation. It found that the fertility window lasts precisely six days, ending on the day of ovulation. As long as intercourse happened inside that six-day window, the timing had no impact on whether the woman would subsequently miscarry, challenging the supposition that sperm sitting around for, say, five days before ovulation would lead to more miscarriages than sperm deposited on the day the ovary releases the egg. Within the six-day window, "older" sperm function just as effectively as their fresher brethren.

This Wilcox study also conveyed a cautionary note to couples who carefully monitor the date of ovulation to best time their intercourse. A woman can detect ovulation by the spike in her body temperature or a rise in her levels of luteinizing hormone (ovulation predictor tests, now sold at pharmacies, measure levels of this biochemical). Couples who abstain from sex until ovulation *reduce* their chances of becoming pregnant. The researchers also found "scant evidence" that frequent intercourse reduced the potency of sperm, as Hertig and Rock and others posited. Bottom line: more sex leads to more pregnancy.

Wilcox's third *New England Journal* article, published in 1999, determined that implantation typically occurs eight to ten days after ovulation. And the earlier implantation occurred, the better. When a conceptus implanted on the ninth day, Wilcox's team discovered, 13 percent miscarried. Implantation on the tenth day doubled the miscarriage rate to 26 percent. By the eleventh day, more than half failed. After the eleventh day, more than four of every five pregnancies failed.

Embryos that take longer than nine days to attach may be somehow impaired, Wilcox asserted. The limited window of receptivity, he and his colleagues concluded, may function to screen out deficient embryos that have trouble implanting.

But this discovery begs another, ultimately deeper question, which I would have to turn elsewhere to explore: What impairs embryos in the first place? The answer, much of the time, lies at a level that Hertig and Rock's microscopes never would have uncovered.

3

SCRAMBLED EGGS

HAVING A BABY ELUDED MICHELLE AND HER HUSBAND, TWO young professionals who live in the midwestern United States. It took them two years of trying to become pregnant, and then, in a tragedy that remained a mystery, the baby died in utero six weeks shy of Michelle's due date. In July 2002, a short two months after that unimaginable loss, Michelle, twenty-nine, was thrilled when she tested positive on a home pregnancy kit. She quickly phoned her doctor's office, and learned the baby's due date: her husband's birthday. Although they could not understand the reason or rhyme, life, it seemed, had started to make sense again.

At the first doctor's appointment, they took a blood sample to determine her level of human chorionic gonadotropin, which should double every two to three days. At the first few check-ins, the hCG levels looked fine. Then, at seven weeks, Michelle and her husband had an ultrasound, which should have revealed a heartbeat. "I think your timing is off," the ultrasound technician told them. "Let me go get the doctor."

"We knew right away," said Michelle.

The doctor explained that Michelle could wait to let the miscarriage take its course or have a dilation and curettage in the next few days. "I didn't want to wait around," said Michelle, who opted for the D and C.

In November 2002, only six months after suffering a stillbirth, Michelle again tested positive on a home test kit. "My husband and I definitely were more cautious this time," she said. "Pregnancy for us equals heartbreak and disaster." Two visits to the doctor showed hCG levels rising at the proper rate. At the seven-week ultrasound, the technician quickly found a heartbeat. "My husband and I were bawling," said Michelle. The technician appeared puzzled by their strong reaction.

"You don't understand," Michelle explained. "We've lost two babies."

The doctor told them they only had a 5 percent chance of miscarriage.

At ten weeks, in January 2003, the doctor checked for a heartbeat with the Doppler, assuring them that if she did not find one, it did not mean the baby had died. Sure enough, the doctor did not find a heartbeat. So she sent them upstairs, where an ultrasound technician would do a finer search for the heartbeat. They walked up the staircase, eyes welling, throats lumpy.

"No heartbeat," the technician coldly told them. "Looks like this baby stopped growing at eight and a half weeks. Sorry." The technician walked out of the room.

"We were just holding each other, bawling again, thinking, What is going on here?"

Again, Michelle chose a D and C, but this time, instead of discarding the slurry of blood and tissue, the doctor dispatched it to the lab in hopes of recovering a piece of fetal or placental tissue for chromosome analysis. Healthy humans have twenty-three pairs of chromosomes, the coiled bundles of DNA that hold our genes. A "karyotype" test isolates the chromosomes found in individual cells and counts them. Karyotyping the tissue from Michelle revealed that this baby had sixty-nine chromosomes, three copies of each one instead of two—a condition called "triploidy," which is not compatible with life. Either Michelle had a bad egg or two sperm had fertilized the same one.

After Michelle's two earlier, inexplicable losses, learning the definitive cause of her miscarriage brought a great sense of relief. "It was nice to know it was abnormal rather than I shouldn't have taken that airplane flight or something," said Michelle. "This one was doomed from conception and was never going to make it. It was nothing I did."

In March 2002, when I first visited Kurt Benirschke in his windowless office next door to the morgue in the basement of the University of California at San Diego (UCSD) Medical Center, he handed me a paper that he had just cowritten about the ovaries of a bottle-nosed dolphin. One of the world's leading authorities on the placenta, Benirschke, then seventy-seven, had had a storied career. After emigrating from Germany to the United States in 1949 with a newly minted M.D., Benirschke worked as a pathologist at Harvard Medical School with Arthur Hertig (then in the middle of his famous early embryo work with John Rock), headed the pathology department at Dartmouth and then UCSD, and, most notably, started the Center for Reproduction of Endangered Species at the San Diego Zoo. He had written or cowritten twenty-nine books, such as the standard *Pathology of the Human Placenta*. He was an expert on the twinning process and birth defects. He had published studies on the genetics of elephants, armadillos, gorillas, marmosets, whales, mules, lemurs, tortoises, cats, bonobos, antelopes, and the Somali wild ass. And his pioneering research linked chromosomal abnormalities to miscarriage.

As Benirschke and I spoke, he juggled a stream of phone calls, other visitors, and regularly turned to check his e-mails, all the while puffing his pipe and filling the air with sweet tobacco smoke. He, too, has a sweetness, a mix of charm, unbounded curiosity, and a mischievous smile. But Benirschke offers his sharp opinions about the ideas and people he has encountered without hesitation or sentiment. Disagree with him, and he'll flap a large hand into the air and say, "Fine, think what you like," and then laugh with a confidence that dares you to ignore this man who, well past the age of retirement for many, continued to devour the scientific literature with the appetite of a graduate student.

Benirschke opened a large box filled with numbered slides standing on edge and took out one that held a miscarried embryo that, like Michelle's baby, possessed three sets of chromosomes. As he showed me the fine points of its abnormalities, it seemed obvious to link miscarriage to odd numbers of chromosomes. But fifty years ago, geneticists did not even know what a normal set of chromosomes looked like.

A 1956 study proved that humans have forty-six chromosomes, two of which determine whether a person is female or male. It took three years before researchers discovered that Down syndrome resulted from three copies—a trisomy—of chromosome 21. The next year, scientists reported that trisomies of chromosomes 13 and 18 explained even more severe maladies. Both typically lead to death within the first year. Benirschke and, independently, David Carr from the University of Western Ontario in Canada both surmised that if these chromosomal abnormalities led to severe health problems and early death, maybe other genetic oddities would explain miscarriage. "No one at the time knew what spontaneous abortions were due to," said Benirschke.

In 1961, a few reports appeared about spontaneous abortions with triploid chromosomes, and at a scientific meeting that year, Benirschke discussed with Carr the possibilities of systematically examining miscarriages for chromosomal errors. By 1963, both had published evidence that aberrations frequently occurred in miscarriages. Of the forty-five miscarriages that Carr and Benirschke karyotyped, they found that almost one in four had chromosomal problems.

The frequency and the diversity of the abnormalities opened a new chapter in reproductive biology. "Everyone was very surprised," said Benirschke.

"Where Have All the Conceptions Gone?" asked C. J. Roberts and C. R. Lowe in a mind-stretching Lancet article they published in 1975. By combining the Hertig and Rock findings with several studies that then had analyzed the frequency of chromosomal abnormalities and miscarriage, Roberts and Lowe concluded that miscarriage occurred far more often than people recognized. And they asserted that many of these losses happened for a good reason. "The notion of controlling the problem of severe malformation at birth by early recognition and abortion is so good and so simple that one wonders why Nature did not think of it first," they wrote. "We believe she did. There is now good evidence that product rejection by way of implantation failure and spontaneous abortion is her principal method of quality control." They went so far as to suggest that "prenatal elimination may perhaps be the rule rather than the exception," a hypothesis they tested with a highly speculative mathematical model.

Drawing on the government registries in England and Wales, Roberts and Lowe tabulated that all the married women there between twenty and twenty-nine years old had approximately 500,000 births and stillbirths in 1971. They compared this figure to a theoretical one they calculated based on several (specious) scientific assumptions. According to their model, most couples had sex twice a week, did not use birth control one out of every four times, and had just a two-day window of fertility. Sperm supposedly fertilized the egg in half of the encounters. All told, these women should have had 2.26 million babies, not 500,000, leading them to conclude that miscarriages occurred with four of every five conceptions.

This provocative study included an equally bold commentary about the significance of their findings. "They are probably not unlike the implications of the discovery that the earth was round, not flat," Roberts and Lowe wrote. "For most people life went on much the same except that what was regarded as a serious problem—what happened to ships when they disappeared over the horizon—was no longer a problem, and therefore ceased to be a source of worry."

Then, five months later, in August 1975, a husband-and-wife team in France, Joëlle and André Boué, working with the statistician Philippe Lazar, offered the first hard evidence that miscarriage occurred much more frequently than commonly believed. In their landmark study, the Boués and Lazar analyzed the karyotypes of almost 1,500 miscarriages, all lost during the first twelve weeks, that they had collected over seven years.

The Boués, like everyone else in this nascent field, stumbled into the study of miscarriage. They worked in Paris at a research center that specialized in polio until the early 1960s, when the success of vaccines against that crippling disease led the entire institution to switch to birth defects. The Boués focused on abnormal embryonic development, which led them to study blood and tissue from pregnancy losses. They contacted ob-gyns throughout Paris, who agreed to give sterile flasks to patients who had the early bleeding or cramping associated with threatened abortions. If the patients miscarried, their doctors asked them to collect any blood and tissue in the flasks. Typically, a woman would have her husband or another person bring the sample directly to the laboratory, which led to a few awkward situations. On one occasion, two different men brought samples from the same woman. "Both of them seemed to be persuaded to be father," remembered Joëlle, noting that they sent the results from their tests to the mother only. "One of the main conditions of medical practice is discretion."

The Boués found that in more than six of every ten miscarriages, the abortus did not have the normal set of twenty-three pairs of chromosomes. As Benirschke and Carr had found, trisomies accounted for more than half of these abnormalities. One in five had three copies of every chromosome, the triploidy that Michelle experienced. Close behind came monosomies, a condition in which a chromosome is missing its partner. (The remaining problems included the odd-sounding tetraploids, mosaics, and translocations, each of which involves too few or too many chromosomes.)

Questioning the histories of their patients, the Boués found no link between abnormal karyotypes and the use of birth control pills; drugs like Clomid, which are used to induce ovulation; prior pregnancies; or the age of the father. But they found a strong correlation between increasing maternal age and trisomies, as others already had discovered with Down syndrome.

During the next five years, similar large studies took place in Hawaii, Sweden, New York, the United Kingdom, and Japan. Each one frequently found a link between miscarriages and odd numbers of chromosomes, with the average frequency being closer to 50 percent than the 61.5 percent that the Boués had arrived at. But an explanation also surfaced for this discrepancy: the Boués had looked at only the first twelve weeks of pregnancy, when most miscarriages occur because chromosomally abnormal embryos typically die shortly after conception. The important discovery that later miscarriages more frequently have chromosomally normal miscarriages has had a practical impact, too, as it influences how clinicians now deal with patients who repeatedly have second-trimester losses.

Why, precisely, do chromosomal abnormalities cause miscarriages? Too many or too few chromosomes equal haywire genes, and they, in turn, often send garbled messages to embryos and placentas, which as a result do not develop properly, frequently ending a pregnancy before or at implantation. Maybe, for example, the haywire genes miscue the formation of the heart or the placental cells as they perform the critical plugging of the mother's spiral arteries. But then why do babies with certain chromosomal abnormalities, like those that result in Down syndrome, sometimes survive? Benirschke suggested that placental size ultimately may draw the line between viable and nonviable, and that some aberrations may allow just enough growth to support life.

As the mechanisms of miscarriage have come into finer focus, so, too, has science's understanding of why these chromosomal abnormalities happen so frequently, and why they become even more common as a woman ages.

In 1980, Patricia Jacobs, Terry Hassold, and their coworkers at the University of Hawaii pushed the field forward with a richly detailed study of the chromosomes from one thousand miscarriages. Using new techniques, the researchers reported the most precise description yet of the various problems that occur. That same year, Jacobs and Hassold combined their results with a study done by a team of researchers led by Dorothy Warburton at Columbia University in New York City, who similarly had karyotyped more than a thousand miscarriages. The cumulative data, from two radically different populations, beautifully complemented each other and set the miscarriage field on a solid scientific footing.

For the next two decades, Warburton, Jacobs, Hassold, and the scientists who studied with them would consistently produce compelling reports that delved ever deeper into the causes of miscarriage. Each also would become expert in the subject, a breed as rare as white Bengal tigers, which gave them novel insights into the human aspects of miscarriages, as well as some of the most imponderable scientific questions.

I met with Jacobs in June 2003 at her laboratory in Salisbury, England. Jacobs, a Scot with a cutting wit, stressed that she studied chromosomal abnormalities, not miscarriage. "I'll just make a generalized statement: all the literature of reproduction in man is rubbish," she said. Many of the deepest insights about reproduction and genetics come from insects like the fly and mammals like the mouse, which Ph.D. researchers, a club she belongs to, study. In contrast, medical doctors have published many of the studies of reproduction and genetics in humans. "They seem to have completely different standards, different criteria," complained Jacobs. "I'm just appalled."

Jacobs, who was about to retire, launched her career with a startling discovery that, more than forty years later, remained the most important finding she had ever made. In 1958, when she was twenty-three and had published one scientific paper (on chromosomal abnormalities found in the testicles of the praying mantis), she analyzed the chromosomes of a man with Klinefelter syndrome, a condition characterized by long limbs, small testicles, and large breasts. She found that the man had forty-seven, rather than forty-six, chromosomes. No one then had ever convincingly described a mammal with an extra chromosome. She went on summer vacation, convinced that she or her technician had done something wrong. But when she returned and redid the experiment, she found that he indeed had an extra X chromosome.

Researchers knew that the X and Y chromosomes determined a person's gender, but they did not know precisely what defined a male or female. Jacobs's discovery of an XXY man revealed that, in humans, the Y chromosome made the man. "I attribute my success to ignorance," said Jacobs, pointing out that more educated geneticists assumed that because the Y chromosome did not determine the sex of a fly, the same held true in humans.

In 1972, Jacobs moved to the University of Hawaii and studied miscarriage because abortuses provided an easy source of genetic abnormalities. Half of miscarriages had chromosomal abnormalities and half did not, which led Jacobs, like the Boués, to recognize that this tidy division presented a natural experiment to tease out the factors that caused these problems. Only one factor clearly explained the cause of trisomy, the main chromosomal abnormality: increasing maternal age. Race had no impact on anything. Women who previously had had an "elective abortion" did not miscarry chromosomally normal babies any more frequently, adding further weight to an earlier finding by Warburton's group that elective abortion does not increase a woman's risk of miscarrying in the future.

One of the study's most revolutionary components had little to do with science: the researchers counseled the women who had miscarried. "We were so horrified by the information given to these women," said Jacobs. "They were being told such appalling things, like miscarriage was extremely rare. They all felt blighted by God. We were telling them something different from their ob-gyns, and we were right. We said, quite the contrary, miscarriage is very common. Go back and ask your mom. Ask your husband's mother. Ask your sisters. Ask the lady next door. At least one, if not all, had had a miscarriage."

I asked Jacobs why she thought humans had such an extraordinarily high miscarriage rate. "It may be partly because we live too long," she said. As women age, she emphasized, they have more difficulty carrying to term, and not just because of increasing chromosomal abnormalities: older women more frequently miscarry normal karyotypes, too. Or maybe, she said, miscarriage occurs frequently for evolutionary reasons, because "our offspring need such huge amounts of parental attention" that fewer children makes families more fit.

Dorothy Warburton, who continues to do miscarriage research at Columbia University, offered a similar answer, suggesting it might provide "a method of child spacing." Like Jacobs, Warburton emphasized that this idea was pure speculation. But it intrigued me that two of the world's most experienced researchers into this subject arrived at the same hypothesis. "We ideally have one child at a time with a very long rearing period," said Warburton, who has the bemused demeanor of an eccentric, wildly intelligent aunt. "I like to joke it's thirty-five years until they get a job."

Many mysteries still surround miscarriage, the creation of abnormal numbers of chromosomes—"aneuploidy"—in particular. "Aneuploidy is the most important problem in human reproduction," Terry Hassold told me. "It's unquestionably the most common genetic problem our species has, and we don't have a clue why it happens."

Benirschke offered a plainspoken, simple explanation. "We don't screw at the right time," he asserted. Consider how other species time their mating, Benirschke said. He offered the example of chimpanzees, our closest relatives. When female chimps ovulate—the process of estrus, or going into heat—their genital area visibly swells. Mating typically occurs at maximal swelling. Humans have no such mechanism, leading to a situation in which many sperm might meet "overripe" eggs that are already disintegrating.

Benirschke, who for eleven years ran the San Diego Zoo's Center for Reproduction of Endangered Species, has as broad a view of pregnancy loss in the animal kingdom as perhaps any living scientist. "If miscarriage happens in other species, it must be quite rare," he said.

Some scientific evidence supports the overripe hypothesis, and some evidence contradicts it. But regardless of why humans miscarry so frequently, researchers over the past two decades have made great strides detailing *how* it happens. "My holy grail is to deliver some sort of pill to reduce aneuploidy," said Hassold, who, with his wife, Patricia Hunt, another Jacobs understudy, later established themselves at Case Western Reserve University in Cleveland, as two of the world's leading researchers on the mechanisms of miscarriage. "The difficulty here is there are a number of routes to aneuploidy. Naïvely, ten, fifteen years ago, I hoped there'd be one major cause."

As studies by Hassold, Hunt, and others have shown, a woman's underlying biology causes 90 percent of the miscarriages that occur because of an extra (trisomy) or a missing (monosomy) chromosome. The eggs of the female fetus each contain two copies of each chromosome for a total of forty-six. The biological cleaver known as meiosis halves these chromosomes, so each at fertilization contains only twenty-three. By combining with the twenty-three ferried in by a sperm cell, it creates a conceptus with forty-six. Actually, meiosis begins when the embryo first makes her eggs — but then the music abruptly stops, "arresting" the forty-six chromosomes in place, until some lucky egg ovulates and meets a sperm. In effect, then, an egg must wait at least a decade and usually several decades to excise and scuttle twenty-three of the chromosomes that it has held since formation. Aneuploidy happens when the process fails to "disjoin" the chromosomes properly, most commonly leaving the about-to-be-fertilized egg with twenty-two or twenty-four chromosomes.

Contrast this process to that in males. The embryonic male makes the precursors to the sperm cells he will one day ejaculate. But unlike the ever depleting original batch of eggs, these so-called spermatogonia, each of which contains forty-six chromosomes, constantly replenish themselves through mitosis, a cousin of meiosis that results in clones that have the same number of chromosomes. At puberty, meiosis kicks in, with batches of spermatogonia regularly diminishing their chromosomes to twenty-three a few months before release.

In an experiment that echoes Hertig and Rock's work, Patricia Hunt investigated the link between age and meiotic errors, helping to clarify the mechanisms that go awry. Hunt and her coworkers harvested eggs from women who had hysterectomies, as well as from women who had had their fallopian tubes tied. The women ranged in age from eighteen to fifty-five. By maturing these eggs in test tubes, Hunt's lab induced them to enter meiosis. They then put fluorescent "tags" on the chromosomes—much like putting a glow stick around a child's neck on Halloween—so they could see the "spindle," the apparatus that pulls them apart, under special microscopes.

The spindle resembles the spinning device from which it takes its name, but only slightly. As the somewhat psychedelic fluorescent photos taken through the microscope show, the oval-shaped spindle looks more like an egg-shaped cobweb of discrete, taut threads. During meiosis, the forty-six chromosomes move from the center down the threads and out to the poles. If all goes well, twenty-three arrive at each end.

Hunt found that for women aged thirty-five or older, about seven out of every ten eggs had odd features: either their chromosomes did not align properly on the spindle threads, or the spindles themselves appeared contorted. Only about one of every ten eggs coming from younger women had similar problems. In all, she found that eggs from older women failed to segregate chromosomes into equal groups at twice the frequency of the young group.

Hunt, who published this study in 1998, said she does not understand the evolutionary logic that would lead females to arrest meiosis from the time they form their eggs and restart it at fertilization. "It strikes me as dangerous to do," she said.

This is the point at which human biology becomes particularly weird—and particularly interesting.

When the twenty-three male chromosomes slip into the downy bed of the egg to make genetic nooky, they pair off with their twenty-three female counterparts, snuggle up to each other, grabbing each other's limbs here and there, and swap similar pieces of DNA. Robert G. Edwards, the British geneticist who created the first test tube baby, cowrote a 1968 study that made a most unusual assertion about chromosomal sex: for meiosis to proceed without error, the male and female chromosomes have to touch each other in many places—and it matters where they touch, too.

In studies of mouse eggs, Edwards and Alan Henderson, both then with the University of Cambridge, found that in older eggs, chromosomes had fewer points at which they touch their partners, and their unions more often occur near the tips. Subsequent studies have verified their basic findings, with one major exception. The frequency of the crossovers and their location does not appear to be linked to age. So what gives?

In 1996, studies from two research groups, coming at the question from radically different perspectives, offered a new, intriguing hypothesis to explain the situation. In one group, fly geneticists studied the X chromosome of Drosophila melanogaster. The other group, which included Terry Hassold, examined Down syndrome in people. Both found that the chromosome pairs with either a reduced number of crossovers or ones that occurred near their tips became more susceptible to sticking together. But whether they actually do stick together—ultimately leading to an egg that contributes either too few or too many chromosomes—depends on age.

In a young woman, the researchers concluded, this increased susceptibility does not necessarily cause problems because the actors that complete meiosis—the spindle apparatus and other players—carry out their assigned roles. Younger eggs have a strong, healthy cast of stagehands that can separate even funky chromosomes. But as eggs age and the stagehands begin to stumble, susceptible chromosomes have more difficulty separating.

R. Scott Hawley, the researcher who headed the fly work, stressed to me that while meiosis fails to pry apart chromosome pairs more frequently as women age, focusing on age itself as the cause actually clouds the picture. "It's not how old the woman is," said Hawley, a geneticist at the Stowers Institute for Medical Research in Kansas City, Missouri. "It's how close she is to menopause."

This distinction matters. As noted earlier, menopause occurs when a woman has roughly a thousand eggs left. Yes, the number of eggs decline as the years pass, and the average age at which menopause begins is fifty-one. But eggs decrease for each woman by her own clock, which means that normal, healthy women can deplete their supply anywhere between forty and sixty years of age.

As Hawley and others contend, the size of the "pool" of eggs determines whether chromosome pairs properly separate because hormones in females control meiosis. And the cells surrounding the eggs secrete hormones. When the egg number declines too low, so do the levels of hormones needed to support the menstrual cycle, triggering menopause. Similarly, the lower levels of hormones affect the timing of the formation of the spindle or other meiotic events, causing what Hawley has jokingly referred to as separation anxiety. "If something's wrong, if that spindle is completed too late or too early, the consequences are going to be failure," said Hawley.

In biomedicine, basic research findings often fail to translate into clinical practice for a myriad of illogical reasons. Assessing the chromosomes in a miscarriage with a karyotype test is a case in point.

W. Allen Hogge, an ob-gyn at Magee-Womens Research Institute at the University of Pittsburgh, first thought that karyotyping each abortus wasted money. But now he argues that, under certain circumstances, karyotyping can save money at a clinic like his—and he has evidence to prove it.

Hogge conducted his own cost-effectiveness study of karyotyping miscarriages from women who had repeated losses. On average, if a woman had recurrent miscarriages, Magee-Womens would spend between $3,000 and $4,000 on various tests to try to determine a root cause of the problem. Karyotyping an embryo or fetus, in contrast, costs no more than $600.

After analyzing 370 cases that miscarried before thirteen weeks, Hogge and his coworkers found that almost seven out of ten had abnormal karyotypes. This relatively high rate in part reflected that a substantial portion of this population was older than thirty-five, when aneuploidy becomes more common. Also, as in the Boué study, the researchers skewed their findings toward more abnormalities by eliminating older fetuses, which women carry further mainly because these babies *rarely* have chromosomal errors. To Hogge, this result meant that only women who miscarried babies with normal karyotypes—less than one-third of his population—needed the battery of expensive (often uncomfortable) tests that clinicians use with recurrent miscarriage patients.

Hogge's analysis had another intriguing finding about women who repeatedly miscarry. Like all pregnant women, these patients often lost chromosomally abnormal babies. "Initially you do not expect that much bad luck for someone," said Hogge. (The odds indeed do change at five or more miscarriages; this unfortunate group of women does lose normal babies at a higher rate.) So for women who have two, three, or even four miscarriages, frequently chance, rather than some underlying biological problem, appears to explain their losses. Indeed, in study after study, women who have up to four miscarriages and become pregnant again typically carry to term.

Women who have had a single miscarriage—by far, the most common situation—face hardly any increased risk of a second loss: a huge study of Danish hospital records looked at 300,000 clinically recognized pregnancies and found that women had an 11 percent risk of miscarrying if they had never had a loss, and it went up to only 16 percent in those who had had a previous miscarriage.

On the other end of the spectrum, a study done by clinicians at St. Mary's Hospital in London, which runs the world's largest recurrent miscarriage clinic, found remarkably high success rates with 201 women who had no identified underlying problem but had each recorded between three and thirteen miscarriages. As the clinic director, Lesley Regan, and her colleagues published in 1997, nearly 70 percent of these women eventually carried to term without any interventions to prevent a miscarriage. (A previous live birth had no impact on the success rate.) Women forty or older did miscarry more frequently (52 percent)—other studies in fact have shown that age matters more than miscarriage history—as did women who had had five or more losses (48 percent). Still, the message gives hope to most everyone who has loved an embryo or a fetus and lost it.

· · ·

In a tony Vancouver, Canada, neighborhood that features expansive homes framed by huge trees and glorious gardens, the Children and Women's Health Centre of British Columbia occupies four square blocks. The rambling complex, which works in collaboration with the University of British Columbia, includes a leading recurrent miscarriage clinic, as well as a large genetics lab that analyzes the chromosomal makeup of some eight hundred "products of conception" each year. Mary Stephenson, the ob-gyn who runs the clinic, stressed that the medical profession must more aggressively mesh state-of-the-art science with miscarriage care. "These patients have been left at the sidelines for so many years," Stephenson told me, noting that she takes particular umbrage at the many studies that lump together women who have trouble getting pregnant with those who have difficulty carrying to term. "We knew so very little ten years ago. And the patients are so appreciative that someone is listening to them."

One of the loudest things miscarriage patients are saying is that they much appreciate knowing whether a chromosomal abnormality caused their loss. "Patients need to know why losses occur," said Stephenson, who has made karyotyping miscarriages a central part of her work.

Karyotyping also has taken on an extra importance for demographic reasons: as more women with what doctors call "advanced maternal age" —thirty-five or older—try to have babies, more chromosomally abnormal miscarriages logically will occur. An analysis by Wendy Robinson, a colleague of Stephenson's who studies meiosis and miscarriage, documented the scale of this demographic shift, charting the changing age of mothers in British Columbia over a three-decade period. In 1968, fewer than 2 percent of the group of women who gave birth for the first time were thirty-five or older, and this age bracket accounted for just over 8 percent of all births. By 2001, 13 percent of first births occurred in the thirty-five-plus group, and it took credit for nearly 20 percent of all births.

Most miscarriages examined in the Vancouver lab rely on tissue removed by the surgical dilation-and-curettage procedure, but the clinic also gives each pregnant patient an eighty-millimeter plastic container, latex gloves, and instructions so that the women can collect whatever blood and tissue they find on their pads or in the toilet bowl. "They feel empowered by doing this," said Stephenson. "We teach them how to educate their doctors. They'll go to emergency rooms and tell them what to do with it."

Karyotyping techniques have changed little in forty years. I accompanied Stephenson to the lab, where Brenda Lomax, the technician who runs it, gave a tour. Several computer monitors in the lab's main room were filled with microscopic images of chromosomes, which from a distance look like dancing stick figures and up close resemble a jumble of caterpillars. Lomax removed from an incubator a petri dish that held a broth of cells freshly isolated from miscarriage material. "The heart stops but the cells keep growing," explained Stephenson. That makes it possible to interrupt the mitotic process at just the right moment and fish out a whole set of separated chromosomes. Staining the chromosomes allows researchers to see them under a microscope.

To the trained eye, an abnormal karyotype "just jumps out at you," said Lomax. "We know the chromosomes like you know your family."

Traditional karyotyping techniques have a few serious drawbacks. Sometimes, the samples are what Lomax called "poor growers," which do not yield sufficient chromosomal information. A mother's cells also often contaminate a sample. Because of the intimate contact between a mother's cells and those from the placenta—or because of the way a D and C can blend macerated embryonic and fetal material with uterine tissue—maternal cells can overgrow the culture. The resultant karyotype will unwittingly isolate the mother's chromosomes by mistake, wrongly leading a clinician to conclude that a patient miscarried a normal female.

Lomax displayed a relatively new method adopted from cancer research which avoids these problems because it does not require growing cells. Called "comparative genomic hybridization," this technique first requires extracting DNA—the material that makes up the chromosomes—and tagging it with a green fluorescent probe. Lomax then takes a sample of DNA from a person she knows has normal chromosomes and labels it with a red fluorescent probe. In the last step, she mixes the red- and green-labeled DNA together and shoots them at the same target, which consists of chromosomes from another normal person. DNA sticks to DNA. If more green than red sticks to the targeted chromosome, a trisomy exists. Another technique allows researchers to quantify the amount of DNA in a sample, further allowing them to detect aberrations that involve complete duplication of the entire set of chromosomes.

Lomax, working with the University of British Columbia's Dagmar Kalousek, in 2000 cowrote a study that documented how profoundly comparative genomic hybridization could affect miscarriage results. Using both this new technique and the old one, the researchers analyzed 301 miscarriage samples. More than one out of every ten samples did not grow well enough for the standard karyotyping. Of the samples that grew successfully, twelve of them were contaminated with maternal cells, leading to an inaccurate karyotype using the conventional technique. In contrast, only six samples lacked enough material to extract DNA for comparative genomic hybridization.

These findings have far-reaching consequences for Stephenson's patients. Lomax drove the point home when she downloaded graphs to her computer screen which represented a sample she just subjected to comparative genomic hybridization. "This is one of Mary's patients that failed to grow, and now we're going to get to the bottom of it," said Lomax. Chromosome 2 clearly had more green than red. "The test sample has an extra copy of 2," Lomax announced. Stephenson, looking over Lomax's shoulder, said that because this patient miscarried an abortus with three copies of chromosome 2, she may not have an underlying problem that requires further tests or interventions.

Stephenson also uses the karyotype information from miscarriages to separate patients in her studies of interventions that aim to prevent miscarriage. She complained that the vast majority of researchers who study recurrent miscarriage do not do so, simply enrolling patients without analyzing the chromosomes of their previous losses. This missed step invariably leads investigators to unwittingly compare patients who have underlying problems to those who do not. "Patient selection is the be all, end all," said Stephenson.

As far back as 1938, Percy Malpas recognized this dilemma. Malpas, a surgeon at the Liverpool Women's Hospital—which, interestingly, today runs one of the few miscarriage clinics in the world—examined the results of two thousand pregnancies, analyzing the frequency of miscarriages. In "A Study of Abortion Sequences," published in the *Journal of Obstetrics and Gynaecology of the British Empire*, Malpas described how he separated patients who miscarried repeatedly from those who had a "spontaneous cure." Malpas reviewed the popular treatments of the day —vitamin E, progesterone, wheat germ oil, iron supplements, and even arsenic—and noted that no studies properly factored in the rate at which untreated women would carry to term. "If the results of any therapy are to be assessed correctly, this question of the spontaneous cure-rate must receive full consideration," wrote Malpas.

Malpas wrote that 18 percent of all pregnancies miscarried, with 17 percent of the losses occurring in women who had no underlying problem and 1 percent in women who had "recurrent losses." So even if a study somehow could focus on these "recurrent aborters," and even if the tested therapy corrected their underlying problem 100 percent of the time, Malpas reasoned that a trial of any intervention should have a miscarriage rate of at least 17 percent. "Results better than this prove too much," he wrote archly.

Malpas recognized a critical truth. But his study—which informed the medical community for decades—proved badly flawed. He vastly overestimated the failure rate of women who repeatedly miscarry—he put it at 73 percent after three losses and 94 percent after four—because he wrongly assumed that any woman who repeatedly miscarried had an underlying problem that would threaten every pregnancy.

In 2002, Stephenson's group published a report that underscored how much diversity exists in any group of women who have recurrently miscarried. The study looked at 285 women who had miscarried between three and twelve times. Just under half of the 420 specimens they karyotyped had an abnormal set of chromosomes, which highlighted that repeated losses often do not mean that the women or their partners have anything fundamentally wrong with their body. The study also offered a fascinating glimpse at the relationship between chromosomal error and age. Women in the eighteen-to-thirty-five age group repeatedly lost chromosomally normal miscarriages 64 percent of the time. In women who were forty or older, the same percentage of miscarriages had *abnormal* chromosomes. So an unidentified biological problem may lurk behind two-thirds of the younger women's miscarriages, but only one-third of the older group's. "The most important thing is to identify patients who have chromosomally normal, recurrent miscarriages," said Stephenson.

Outside of recurrent miscarriage centers and the few cost-conscious clinicians, like Allen Hogge, who work at fertility centers or more generalized prenatal clinics, few practitioners to this day will do a chromosomal analysis of patients' miscarriages, despite the insistence of experts like Stephenson that it plays an essential role in determining how to address losses.

In September 2003, I checked in with Michelle, the woman in the Midwest who had had a stillbirth at thirty-four weeks and two subsequent miscarriages, one of which proved to have triploidy. "I am 7 mos pregnant and hoping and praying for a great outcome this time!" she e-mailed me. "We are having a boy and I'm being watched closely by a high risk group, so HOPEFULLY my story will have a nice ending!" Michelle acknowledged that she in fact already had tested positive when we last spoke in late March, but she didn't want to say anything. "You know how that is!"

On November 20, thirty-seven weeks pregnant, doctors induced her. "My nerves couldn't go much longer," she said. Michelle delivered a healthy boy.

PART TWO

MYSTERIES

4

REJECTION

By the time Jess agreed to receive injections of her husband's white blood cells, she had endured the cycle of hope and heartbreak that torments many women who seek medical help to conceive and carry a child to term. Jess, a friend who lives in southern California and asked that I refer to her by nickname only, began her odyssey into the world of reproductive medicine at twenty-nine, when her gynecologist diagnosed her with endometriosis. Two surgeries took care of this problem, which involves removing uterine-like tissue that for some reason grows outside the uterus and can lead to irregular bleeding, ovarian cysts, and inflammation and scarring of the fallopian tubes. But even with the surgeries, her gynecologist warned that she might have trouble becoming pregnant. So at the relatively young age of thirty-two, Jess and her husband saw their first of many fertility specialists.

Jess soon began taking Clomid to stimulate the ovaries to produce more eggs. No luck. Less than a year later, she tried in vitro fertilization and embryo transfer. "The whole experience was a complete disaster," recalled Jess, a strong, soft-spoken woman whose emotions often are overshadowed by her intensely rational approach to matters. "I knew as soon as they put it in—it all ran out." Next, Jess and her husband consulted the same renowned clinician whom Shannon and I once visited. A few weeks later, while still in the midst of a workup with the new doctor, Jess learned she was pregnant.

Jess waited until she was in her third month to tell her parents the good news. The next month—just as with Shannon, on a Labor Day weekend—cramping prompted her to phone her doctor. "She told me, 'Well, there's nothing I can do,'" remembered Jess. At 5 A.M. the next morning, she miscarried. "I went to the bathroom and it was a baby with eyes and arms," Jess said. "We were both pretty much a mess. I didn't shed any tears before any of this happened."

They put the fetus in Tupperware, refrigerated it, and toted it to the doctors the next day for analysis. But lab technicians mishandled the sample. "They botched it," she said. A doctor at the clinic had some advice for Jess's husband. "Don't read anything," he said. "It's just going to confuse you."

After doing extensive research on the Internet, Jess identified the California clinic that had the highest IVF success rate for women in her age bracket who had endometriosis: San Francisco's Pacific Fertility Center. In March 1998, seven months after her miscarriage, she and her husband met with one of that center's doctors, who said she could decrease the risk of miscarriage by receiving injections of her husband's white blood cells, or lymphocytes. After more research, Jess had only a vague understanding of why lymphocyte immune therapy might help, but she agreed. "I knew they were suggesting things that I hadn't seen elsewhere," said Jess. "I didn't read anything that said, 'No, stop.' That's what I was looking for. They had a good record at their clinic, and I took a leap of faith."

Proponents of lymphocyte immune therapy contend that it prevents miscarriage much as a vaccine prevents disease. The idea rests on the supposition that a woman can have an aberrant immune response to her baby, which, because of the contribution of the father's genes, looks like a trespasser. Injecting the father's white blood cells into the mother theoretically will make her immune system more tolerant of the foreigner.

Huge controversies surround lymphocyte immune therapy. Supporters portray the treatment as cutting-edge science. Detractors see it as something akin to voodoo, and stress that carefully done studies have shown that it does not work and may even *increase* the risk of miscarriage. Despite the noisy debates, many couples plug their ears and firmly believe that because of the treatment, they have babies—and no amount of scientific data can shake the power of that conviction.

The notion that immune reactions cause many miscarriages dates back to 1952, when the British immunologist Peter Medawar attended a meeting on evolution and gave a lecture—published the next year in what became a landmark paper—that asked why a mother routinely did not reject a fetus. Brazilian born and Oxford educated, Medawar, at six feet five inches, stood tall both literally and figuratively, pioneering the nascent field of transplant biology. Scientists long had known that if you transplanted skin or an organ from one animal to another, the immune system of the recipient would attack this graft, destroying it within weeks. The immune system regarded the foreign graft as a dangerous intruder, like a virus or bacteria, that it had to eliminate swiftly. This process of rejection helped establish the idea that the immune system distinguishes "self," which it knows not to attack, from "nonself." Medawar viewed the fetus as a graft. This concept has profoundly influenced, at one point or another, most every leading researcher who has studied miscarriage.

Medawar's lecture had a range as expansive as its title: "Some Immunological and Endocrinological Problems Raised by the Evolution of Viviparity in Vertebrates." Viviparity, the ability for a mother to carry offspring and birth a live baby, marked an evolutionary giant step from egg-laying birds, reptiles, and fish, and it profoundly changed the relationship between mother and child. Medawar, reminiscent of Kurt Benirschke, had a vast knowledge of different species. In a tone that alternated between ponderous and mystified, Medawar took a deep dive into the question of why the immune systems of viviparous mothers did not immediately give the boot to every offspring, a clump of rapidly dividing cells that resembled a tumor. He acknowledged that his ideas were "highly speculative, and may turn out to be very much mistaken," stressing that "even if we set down all the known causes of antenatal mortality or miscarriage, the unexplained residue is of stirring proportions."

The unexplained residue led Medawar to review the discovery, first made in 1939, that a mother could have an immunologic reaction against her own fetus. The finding came about after a twenty-five-year-old woman gave birth to a stillborn fetus and then received a transfusion from her husband, who shared her blood type. The woman had a transfusion reaction, in which her immune system savaged the donated blood cells, leading to the suspicion that the fetus had inherited something from the father that the mother's immune system similarly had attacked.

Subsequent work the next year revealed that "something": a protein, first discovered in the rhesus monkey, that exists in roughly 85 percent of Caucasians, 90 percent of blacks, and 99 percent of Asians. As it soon became clear, when a mother *does not* have the so-called Rh factor and conceives a child with a man who *does* have the Rh factor, the baby often will be Rh-positive, and its blood can trigger an antibody reaction in her. This antibody response is relatively weak with a first child. But for a pregnant, Rh-negative women who has had a child or a miscarriage, her immune responses can kill the baby. This discovery, Medawar said, "is one of the triumphs of modern clinical biology."

But Medawar had less interest in the relatively rare Rh incompatibility (now easily treated) than he did in the principle it illustrated, which he thought should apply to every pregnancy. From the perspective of the immune system, each person has a unique "bar code," which appears as an array of proteins—known as antigens—on the surface of each cell. Although scientists in 1952 had only a rudimentary idea of how the immune system uses these bar codes to distinguish self from nonself, Medawar understood that a mother's antigens had to differ from those in her fetus, which of course had a mix of maternal and paternal genes. Then, why, he wondered, doesn't every mother launch an immune attack against her own fetus? Medawar cautioned that "it would be most unwise to overlook the possibility" that when a mother's immune system sees this nonself jumble of antigens in the fetus, it may attack and cause a miscarriage, "particularly in the early stages of pregnancy."

Medawar laid out three possible reasons that this reaction might not occur. Maybe a barrier separated the fetal and maternal circulation. Maybe the fetus had such immature antigens that the mother's immune system did not recognize it as foreign. Or maybe the mother's immune system becomes inert to the foreigner and tolerates its presence.

The idea of tolerance built on an experiment that Medawar and his coworkers had just completed. Intrigued by the finding that fraternal (nonidentical) twin calves often have a mixture of each other's red blood cells, Medawar's team in 1951 reported that they could graft skin from one fraternal calf twin to another. Somehow, it seemed, because these chimerical calves had the foreign cells in them from birth, their immune systems had become tolerant of the skin of their siblings. Medawar's lab then took this experiment a step further, demonstrating that they could artificially make a mouse tolerant of another mouse's cells by injecting the foreign cells into a fetal or newborn mouse.

Medawar proposed that maybe a pregnant woman or her fetus produced increased levels of cortisone, a hormone that researchers had discovered could dampen immune reactions to grafts. Scant evidence supported the idea, which even he downplayed as "merely thinking aloud." But the question he raised remained: Did something rein in a pregnant woman's immune system to prevent it from rejecting her baby?

Medawar's musings unintentionally spawned the field of reproductive immunology, which has searched high and low for evidence that immune reactions can cause miscarriages—and for treatments that can redirect the aberrant response. Medawar, who in 1960 won the Nobel Prize for helping to discover the fundamental finding that allows surgeons to graft skin onto burn victims and transplant kidneys, hearts, and other organs, ironically did not study reproductive immunology. But, as early as 1963, his erstwhile graduate student and frequent coauthor, Rupert Billingham, investigated the idea of the fetus as a transplant.

In a two-part paper that ran so long that the *New England Journal of Medicine* published it in back-to-back issues in 1964, Billingham picked up the discussion where Medawar left off. He rejected the idea that the fetus lived in some immune-privileged site that remained impervious to attack because of some sort of barrier. Not only did blood cells clearly pass between mother and fetus, as the Rh-factor indicated, but many experiments in animals confirmed that cells could cross the placenta in either direction. New information, some of it from Billingham's own lab, "decisively refuted" Medawar's second thesis that said the embryo or young fetus had yet to produce the antigens capable of triggering an immune response. Only one possibility remained: the mother's immune system, by some unknown mechanism, tolerated the fetus.

Yet Billingham also presented a compelling argument to trash Medawar's idea about cortisone-inducing tolerance. If pregnancy increased cortisone, then pregnant women should better tolerate foreign grafts. In experiments with skin grafts put on mice and cattle, pregnancy did nothing to abate the immunologic attack on the foreign material. Years would pass before Billingham put forward his own theory about maternal immunologic tolerance. And it would become the intellectual rationale for lymphocyte immune therapy, the unusual miscarriage treatment tried by Jess and thousands of other women.

The imprimatur of the *New England Journal* legitimizes ideas in the medical world. In the world of basic research, *Science*, started by Thomas Edison, is one of the few journals that has similar, if not greater, powers. In 1973, *Science* published a groundbreaking study on pregnancy and haywire maternal immunity by Billingham, then at Southwestern Medical School in Dallas, and Alan Beer, an ob-gyn resident. In rat experiments, Billingham and Beer showed for the first time that they could create a disease in offspring by artificially biasing the mother's immune system against paternal antigens in a mother's own pups. They then showed that they could use the paternal antigens to, in effect, immunize a female such that she would not attack her pup for having some of its father's genes. Specifically, they theorized that their immunization created "blocking antibodies" in the mother that prevented her white blood cells from harming the pup. So they used the immune system to stop the immune system.

Between 1970 and 1980, Billingham and Beer would explore these ideas extensively in animal experiments, publishing two dozen articles together, none of which appeared in journals as discriminating as *Science*, although one, "The Embryo as a Transplant," ran in the widely read *Scientific American*. By 1975, their thinking took a sharp, surprising turn. Studies in mice, hamsters, and rats led them to conclude that, as they wrote in one paper, "genetic disparity between a conceptus and its mother significantly improves its chances of implantation and development to term." Genetic *disparity*?

Yes, Billingham and Beer had found that the *more* genetically dissimilar the parents, the better the chance the mother would carry to term. This finding represented a significant shift away from the earlier hypothesis that mothers attacked their fetuses *because* of their genetic differences. Owing at least in part to the fuzziness of their data, Billingham and Beer could not explicitly spell out the mechanism behind this new theory, but in essence they had shifted their sights from rejection to protection of the fetus. Essentially, they stuck with their original thesis that the maternal immune system naturally attacks the fetus, but they now contended that the same maternal immune system protected the fetus from this attack—but only if the parents had large enough genetic differences to lead the mother to make "blocking antibodies."

This pretzel logic made some sense, as it confirmed the widely held taboo against inbreeding. But biologists dislike theories that lack clear-cut mechanisms, and from the start, this thesis had question marks stamped all over it. Still, clinical researchers can silence hard-core biologists by testing an intervention based on a murky theory and showing that it works. The history of vaccines provided ample evidence: Edward Jenner successfully showed that immunization could prevent smallpox before scientists had even discovered viruses or the immune system. And, ultimately, if a medical intervention works, the mechanism is academic.

In 1979, Beer put Billingham and Medawar's theory to the test in humans. The study recruited three couples who satisfied the theory's profile. Each had endured between five and seven early miscarriages, and tests of their blood revealed an unusually high genetic similarity between the partners. Beer mixed white blood cells from each couple in test tubes and found that they did not react much, putatively because their similarities prevented the immune responses that typically occur in this experiment. As a result of these women's immune systems tolerating the invasion by their partners, he posited, the women did not produce the blocking antibodies that would protect their fetuses, leading to what he called "reproductive inefficiency." An injection of the partners' white blood cells might overwhelm the all too accepting immune system of the women, "breaking" tolerance by forcing their bodies to make blocking antibodies when confronted with their partners' antigens.

The first woman to become pregnant after treatment with her husband's lymphocytes had experienced seven miscarriages. The thirty-nine-year-old professional found Beer after searching Medline, a National Library of Medicine database, to identify the leading recurrent miscarriage researchers. "I received numerous articles," the woman told me. (She asked that I refer to her by the initials "S.J.," which Beer used in a paper describing her case.) "I didn't even read them until later. I was just looking for those individuals who had the most concentrated research on the subject, and Dr. Beer had four articles more than anyone else."

In the fall of 1979, S.J. met with Beer for the first time at the University of Michigan, where he then worked. At Beer's request, S.J. brought a blood sample from her husband and one of her own. For dramatic effect, she toted them in a diaper bag. "I was trying to get his attention." S.J. laughed, adding, "I have a little ham in me." They spoke for several hours. "He's a very impressive man—very philosophical, very capable, supportive, and informative," she said.

To S.J., Beer represented her last shot at having a child. At her seventh and most emotionally painful miscarriage, she sobbed along with both her husband and her ob-gyn. "All three of us were very, very sad," she remembered some twenty-five years later. "My husband said, 'Enough. We can't do this anymore.'" S.J. sought counseling with her ob-gyn as well. "I was trying to figure out what was the right thing to do, because my husband was very exhausted with the emotional and physical roller coaster we'd been through, and I felt I wanted one more chance," said S.J. Her miscarriages also led her to have a "major discussion with the man upstairs," she said. "I was really trying to ponder if I should proceed one more time."

Shortly after receiving an infusion of her husband's white blood cells, S.J. became pregnant. For her fortieth birthday, her husband commissioned a portrait of their cat atop her pregnant belly. "I loved that picture," she told me. "I thought, If I can't deliver, at least I'll have a portrait of my being pregnant." In September 1980, she gave birth to the first "Beer baby," a healthy six-pound, eight-ounce boy. "I literally see Dr. Beer as a godsend," S.J. said. "He is still a very good friend and, in my opinion, a consummate and caring physician without peer."

Across the Atlantic, James Mowbray, a researcher at St. Mary's Hospital Medical School in London who specialized in transplantation and the immune system, similarly had started to study whether lymphocyte immunization could prevent miscarriages in women who had repeated losses. In the transplantation field, several researchers had shown that they could increase the survival of a graft or organ by first immunizing the recipient with the donor's white blood cells. Extending the concept to miscarriage seemed to make imminent sense.

Mowbray and his coworkers went a step beyond Beer, organizing a carefully designed study that aimed to assess whether the treatment truly worked. Given that many, if not most, pregnant women who have had repeated miscarriages in the past will carry to term with no medical intervention, researchers are hard put to determine whether an intervention works. Say that 50 percent of the women in a study will carry to term without any treatment. A study could prescribe chewing gum to one hundred pregnant women who had had recurrent miscarriages and then claim that the treatment worked half the time.

To circumvent such problems, clinical researchers rely on the "placebo-controlled, double-blind, randomized trial." The researchers first select patients with similar characteristics and then randomly divide them into two groups: one receives the treatment, while the other gets a dummy, or placebo, medication. To reduce biases, the trial remains blinded to both the clinician and the participant, which means neither knows who receives the treatment until the end of the study. In 1982, Mowbray launched the first placebo-controlled, double-blind, randomized trial of lymphocyte immune therapy.

As a sign of their rigor, Mowbray and his coworkers studied 209 women who had had at least three miscarriages with the same partner, and excluded 104 because of such potentially confounding variables as being Rh-negative, already having a detectable antibody against her partner, or having a clear cause for her losses (such as a chromosomal problem in either the man or woman). Of the 105 women who participated in the trial, only 47 became pregnant and completed the study.

Upon becoming pregnant, the women either received injections of lymphocytes from their husbands, or, if they were in the control group, injections of their own white blood cells. As Mowbray and his colleagues reported in *The Lancet* in 1985, 78 percent of the women in the treatment group had a live birth, while only 37 percent in the placebo group carried to term. The researchers concluded that the immunization with paternal cells "produced a highly significantly [sic] better result."

As impressive as those results sound, a study published the year before by a husband-and-wife research team in Norway had similar results by simply offering women "tender-loving care."

Between 1971 and 1980, Babill and Sverre Stray-Pedersen, in Oslo, followed 195 couples who had had three or more miscarriages. After thoroughly evaluating the couples for underlying problems, they determined that 85 had "unknown" causes for their miscarriages. They then separated 61 of these women who became pregnant into two groups. The control group, 24 women, received no treatment. The researchers offered the other 37 women tender-loving care, which consisted of psychological support and weekly medical exams. In the control group, only one-third carried to term. In contrast, 86 percent of the treated women delivered healthy babies.

Mowbray and his coauthors noted the Stray-Pedersen results in the *Lancet* paper that discussed their findings, and indeed the design of their lymphocyte immune therapy study offered similar care to both the treated and untreated groups. Yet the Stray-Pedersen findings until this day call into question any study of drugs or surgery that claim success — Did both a treated and control group receive the same tender-loving care? Did one receive more than the other? Did the groups differ in the tender-loving care they received outside of the study? — and they help explain why heated controversies have dogged lymphocyte immune therapy and most every other attempt to help women carry babies to term. "It's a very muddy pool," Mowbray, who had retired, told me in 2001. "Recurrent abortion is not a state, a condition, or a disease. It's a malfunction. And if it has quite a lot of causes, it will remain a muddy pool."

After his seminal 1985 publication, Mowbray continued to treat women with lymphocyte immunizations, as did Beer and many other clinicians around the world. A 1986 story in *Newsweek* on miscarriage offered lymphocyte immune therapy as an example of recent progress in preventing miscarriage "that is little short of spectacular." The article singled out Beer, reporting that he had immunized 119 women: 96 had conceived, 52 had carried to term, 24 were still pregnant, and only 20 had miscarried. These raw, preliminary, uncontrolled results had no decipherable scientific meaning, nor did the article quote Beer suggesting that they did. But this detail did not faze the *Newsweek* writers, who described Beer's lymphocyte immune therapy as "simple, elegant and overwhelmingly effective."

Randomized, controlled studies soon launched in Australia, Taiwan, Denmark, Italy, Scotland, the United States, and England produced conflicting results, but each one included fewer than a hundred people, making it difficult to arrive at a statistically robust answer to the question of whether lymphocyte immunization helped, did nothing, or even caused harm. By the early 1990s, so much confusion surrounded the intervention that researchers began to lump information from different trials into what researchers call "meta-analyses." Although differences surely exist among studies, a meta-analysis strives to find clarity in a muddy pool by assuming that all patients participated in the same trial, which allows researchers to look at the largest possible number of controlled and treated people. One meta-analysis published in 1993 found that lymphocyte immune therapy did nothing, while the next year, two other reports, sponsored by the American Society for Reproductive Immunology, found a slightly higher success rate in treated (70 percent) versus untreated (60 percent) women.

Mowbray, and many others, looked askance at Beer, one of the most aggressive proponents of the intervention, because he did not publish a double-blind, randomized, placebo-controlled study of his work. "He's never really done a controlled trial in an orderly way, and he tends to shift treatment from patient to patient," Mowbray complained to me. Some also stressed that the treatment potentially presented serious risks. As with any blood transfusion, the procedure could transmit an undetected infection harbored inside the man's blood cells; HIV and hepatitis C both were transmitted unwittingly from blood donors to recipients for several years before science had the tools to detect them. Injections of another person's blood cells also could trigger a dangerous immune reaction similar to what happens when a person rejects a graft. On top of these concerns, Carole Ober, a geneticist at the University of Chicago who specializes in miscarriage, pointed out that there may be risks that scientists cannot even imagine. "People tend to be very cavalier about injecting foreign cells into these women," Ober complained to me. "We don't know what will happen over time."

Ober, like many researchers, tired of the endless debates, organized a study in 1992 that hoped to answer the question once and for all, calming the furor. The Recurrent Miscarriage Study, or REMIS, aimed to recruit 524 couples. The randomized, double-blind, placebo-controlled study planned to enroll patients for four years. At the outset, Alan Beer, who by then had moved to the Chicago Medical School and ran a popular clinic that offered lymphocyte immune therapy, had agreed to participate. Ober was much heartened. "I adored the man," Ober said. "It's because of Alan that I became involved with this field."

By the end of the study, Ober and Beer had what amounted to irreconcilable differences.

On March 6, 1998, three days after a doctor at the Pacific Fertility Center told my friend Jess that lymphocyte immune therapy might help her carry a baby to term, an independent committee known as the Data Safety Monitoring Board recommended that Ober and her coinvestigators—a prominent group that included Mary Stephenson from Vancouver but not, notably, Alan Beer—stop REMIS. Public health regulations in the United States and elsewhere mandate such a monitoring board to serve as the objective outsider in a clinical study, periodically reviewing its progress, and protecting trial participants by stopping an experiment early when the results unequivocally show harm or benefit. Confronted with the revelation that women who received lymphocyte immune therapy had *higher* miscarriage rates than those in the placebo group, the REMIS investigators promptly halted the $2.2 million trial.

The REMIS investigators did not publicize the trial's results for more than a year, nor did the National Institutes of Health, its sponsor, or the Food and Drug Administration, which regulates clinical trials. Across the country, independent practitioners continued to advocate the therapy.

The Pacific Fertility Center referred Jess to the Los Olivos Women's Medical Group in Los Gatos, near San Jose, which performed lymphocyte immune therapy in conjunction with Alan Beer. In September 1998, Jess received the first of three injections. In November, after having received two infusions of her husband's white blood cells, she returned to the Pacific Fertility Center for a transfer of five embryos, and then, later in the month, visited Los Olivos for one more lymphocyte immunization. The next month, Jess learned she was pregnant. "The whole time, everything was wonderful," Jess said.

In August 1999, Jess gave birth to a healthy baby girl.

One month earlier, in the July 31, 1999, issue of The Lancet, Carole Ober, Mary Stephenson, and the other coinvestigators published a full report of the REMIS study. Before the investigators stopped the trial, 171 women who had recurrent miscarriages met the enrollment criteria (at least three miscarriages of unknown cause) and either received the placebo or the treatment. By the end of the study, 68 women in the treatment group had become pregnant and almost half of them carried to term. In the placebo group, 65 percent of the 63 pregnancies ended in a live birth. "Because of the lack of benefit, we recommend against this intervention as a treatment for unexplained recurrent miscarriage," concluded the researchers.

By July 2001, when I first contacted Alan Beer, his reputation for successfully treating miscarriage had spread worldwide. "We've all talked to patients who go there, and they're devoted to the guy," said the ob-gyn James Scott, a REMIS coinvestigator based at the University of Utah who trained with Beer under the pioneering reproductive immunologist Rupert Billingham. People magazine had profiled Beer in a 1996 story headlined "Injection of Hope," which opened with a photograph of the doctor, a white-haired Marcus Welby look-alike, swarmed by a gaggle of infants, toddlers, and children at a "Beer Baby Reunion." Beer also received national attention on the NBC newsmagazine Dateline, which ran a segment on him in 2000.

Beer's Web site described his Reproductive Medicine Program in great detail. Links offered lengthy discussions of lymphocyte immune therapy and various scientific topics. A guide offered tips to those who sought reimbursement from insurance companies for reproductive immunology treatment. Testimonials from patients confirmed that many had a deep devotion that rose to the level of adoration.

One such testimonial came from a husband whose wife had had seven losses. For those struggling with miscarriage, he wrote, Beer was the *only* doctor who could help. "Trust me, I know!!!" the man exclaimed. "This Doctor has the talent of Michael Jordan, the intelligence of Bill Gates, and the love for people in need like Mother Teresa. I say this because he is the first person in our lives (other than our parents) that cared enough about us and wanted to really help us. Dr. Beer is what a Doctor should be like. God bless you Dr. Beer."

Another husband and wife, who carried a daughter, Gabrielle, to term, penned a poem, "One Man—A Tribute to Dr. Beer":

> For all the babies who came and went without ever being born,
> For all the mothers who wept and wept and remained forlorn,
> For all the fathers who felt more helpless year after year,
> For all of them, now and soon, God gave us Dr. Beer!
> One Man who feels enough to understand the pain,
> One Man who knows enough to prevent it from happening again.
> One Man who cares enough to take the time to learn,
> One Man who dares enough to take a different turn.
> One Man who saved us from our living hell—
> One Man—one man—who gave us Gabrielle!!

Headquartered at Chicago Medical School's Finch University of Health Sciences, Beer's program divided immune problems that cause miscarriage into five categories, treating two of them with lymphocyte immune therapy. Beer's "Consumer's Guide" to lymphocyte immune therapy offered one of the most explicit discussions I had read about the mechanism of blocking antibodies, although even it left me scratching my head. "What does blocking antibody do?" the Web site asked. "This question still cannot be answered in its final form. It is believed that the antibody produced by the mother attaches to the cells of the placenta (produced by the father) and camouflages them from rejection by the mother—'making them look like a wolf in sheep's clothing.' In addition, it is believed that this antibody functions as fertilizer to the placenta and provides nourishment that makes it grow and 'root' and attach to the placenta."

One of Beer's sharpest critics, Joseph Hill, who ran the recurrent miscarriage clinic at Harvard Medical School's Brigham and Women's Hospital until going into private practice in 2002, ridiculed the Web site when I spoke with him. "He has a lot of information," Hill said. "Most of it is misinformation. It's a great religion." Hill, like Mowbray, criticized Beer for not conducting rigorous studies of lymphocyte immune therapy and other interventions. "He's quite the salesman," said Hill, who once spent time with Beer to learn from him. "He's very charismatic, and he talks a good game. But he says things when there's no data whatsoever. The sad thing is he's never bothered to test his ideas in a scientific manner. He's the fringe. But he has a large following."

Curious about Beer's claims and intrigued that Beer still offered lymphocyte immune therapy after the REMIS study's negative results, I sent him an e-mail to request an interview. He promptly wrote back a most cordial note. "I am happy to talk to you because I am the Father of reproductive immunology in the US," he wrote. The REMIS study, he contended, "was flawed." During the next few weeks, we spoke at length over the phone, and exchanged several detailed e-mails. According to Beer, he had treated more than twelve thousand women with lymphocyte immune therapy, many of whom simultaneously received other immune-based interventions. His patients were, on average, 38.6 years old, had 4.4 miscarriages, and were "bruised, abused and often without hope." He claimed that 86.9 percent—the decimal-point precision implying that he had carefully measured—of those who received lymphocyte immune therapy gave birth to a live baby. Without treatment, he said, only 25 percent would carry to term.

Looking back on REMIS, Alan Beer stressed that the study never would have happened without his help. And he is right. The National Institutes of Health twice turned down Carole Ober's proposal to stage the REMIS study because of concerns that she could not recruit enough patients. "They said you'll never get patients because Alan Beer is in Chicago," recalled Ober. Indeed, why would a woman, especially one who had concerns about the ticking of her biological clock, join Ober's study, where she might receive a placebo, when she could go across town and receive the treatment from the world-famous Beer?

Ober got her grant in 1992 after Beer agreed to send his patients to the randomized, placebo-controlled study. He also stressed to me that he chaired the peer group that evaluated the grant submission. But Ober and her coworkers charged that Beer never really cooperated after that point. "Toward the end of the second year, it was very clear that Alan was not sending us any patients," Ober said.

Beer explained it differently—and the details of this internecine disagreement went a long way toward helping me understand why so many miscarriage studies have difficulty arriving at scientifically sturdy conclusions. "I had referred one hundred twenty-four documented patients to their screening nurse," he said. "And none of these patients were accepted into the trial or agreed to be randomized. Now one of the problems was that I was accused of biasing the patients because they came to me first expecting consultation with me and treatment, and were given the option of a randomized study. When the nurse counseled them that they could be part of the study, have the testing, and if they failed they could go back to Dr. Beer's program and get the treatment for free, they essentially said, 'Piss off.' And I was blamed for that."

As for the heat Beer has received over the years for not staging randomized, double-blind controlled studies of his many experimental therapies, he agreed that such carefully designed trials would help the field. "I wish that there could be double-blind studies done on all aspects of this," Beer said. "But when you're dealing with the infertile patient, you're dealing with someone who is suspicious, damaged, guarded— who is self-blaming and isn't really interested in a double-blind research study. I didn't realize that when we started this. I never thought that the patients would not agree to be randomized. And that was a huge problem." A few minutes later, he offered an even more dramatic explanation. "When your baby dies inside of your uterus, patients come to me with a different mentality."

But the REMIS investigators *did* find 171 qualified women who volunteered to join the study, so the obstacles, while real, do not present insurmountable hurdles. (More evidence that researchers can clear these hurdles comes from Lesley Regan at St. Mary's in London, whose group has conducted several recurrent miscarriage studies. "I've actually spent a lot of time doing randomized trials," she told me. "I've never had a problem recruiting patients.")

Beer also pointed out that the REMIS researchers fell far short of their original goal of 524 couples, and he contended that the study had to relax its entry criteria to find even those 171 women, possibly allowing in people who had other underlying problems. And he disagreed with the way the REMIS researchers prepared the lymphocytes from the men, claiming that because they typically stored them overnight, the cells had lost their potency. "Even in my hands, the cells would be dead and not beneficial," he said. (James Mowbray similarly made the point to me that he always used fresh cells, and that dead ones did not work.)

Beer went so far as to call the REMIS study "dangerous," stressing that he encourages women to use birth control until they have developed what he deems the proper immune responses to the immunization. REMIS did not do so. "Inadequately treated patients will be made worse, because you can really inflame their immune problem," said Beer. The way REMIS used lymphocyte immune therapy, he asserted, "kills babies."

Debate thrives in every biomedical field. The difference between, say, AIDS and miscarriage research is not in the volume or the passion of the debate, but in the quality. AIDS researchers, as frequently and stridently as they disagree with one another, carry out many studies that yield interpretable results, ending fractious fights. Drugs can prevent transmission of the AIDS virus from mother to baby. Condoms slow epidemics. Specific cocktails of specific drugs can prolong an infected person's life. In the miscarriage arena, no such lingua franca unites the quarrelsome factions, and, at times, it seems as though everyone disagrees about everything, with no amount of data ever ending a debate.

A confluence of factors handicaps miscarriage research. Many interventions, lymphocyte immune therapy among them, have no corporate sponsor, which removes the incentive to design expensive, well-controlled studies that will pass muster at the Food and Drug Administration. Because, as I explained earlier, most women who miscarry up to four times will eventually carry to term without any help, any treatment that does not cause harm will appear effective, regardless of its true merit. And each woman who becomes convinced that something worked for her becomes an advocate for it, which must make it more difficult to recruit people to the randomized, placebo-controlled studies that separate science from anecdote. Finally, the fuzzy scientific rationale behind theories often makes it difficult to select patients who indeed *may* benefit from a treatment.

To try to resolve the lymphocyte immune therapy debate once and for all, I played middleman in the point-counterpoint arguments of Beer and his critics. Ober and her coworkers presented me with rational rebuttals to each criticism. REMIS modeled itself after the 1985 Mowbray study and used precisely the same entry criteria. The investigators did measure immune responses to the immunization, although they did not find that they had any correlation with success or failure. No evidence from other studies showed that fresh cells worked better. Paul Meier, a prominent biostatistician at Columbia University who served on the independent board that monitored and halted the REMIS trial, insisted that the study was "very well done" and said that there was simply no rationale for continuing to offer the treatment.

I ran these rebuttals by Beer, who remained resolute that he could help women carry to term with lymphocyte immune therapy. And the REMIS study, he said, had had no impact on the interest his patients had in the intervention. "Zero," said Beer. "Not a blip on the screen. Which was a huge surprise to me. One can devote your life to something and find out that it was wrong or dangerous or not expected. I think quite the opposite right now. We are now just learning that the lymphocyte immune therapy mimics an individual with normal pregnancy."

The REMIS investigators and other researchers I spoke with who knew the results decried the fact that Beer and others continued to offer lymphocyte immune therapy. "I've been personally amazed that this continues," said James Scott, who, in addition to his role as a REMIS coinvestigator, is editor of the prominent journal *Obstetrics & Gynecology*. Another coinvestigator, James Schreiber, head of the ob-gyn department at the Washington University School of Medicine in St. Louis, allowed that he was convinced that lymphocyte immune therapy did *something*. "But I'm also convinced that it doesn't help someone have a child," Schreiber said. Harvard's Joseph Hill, who did not participate in REMIS, said it was the sixth and best trial to find that the therapy does not work. "I don't understand why it's allowed to remain available," Hill said.

Beer attempted to take the criticisms in stride, but the barbs clearly exasperated him. "I'm talked about as this witch doctor," he said at one point, noting that he had published more than one hundred studies about reproductive immunology. "If I'm wrong, why aren't the patients going to them?" he asked. He went on to explain that his most vocal critics did not have his database of evidence. "Knowing the data that I know, I really pity the critics."

I contacted the Food and Drug Administration to clarify how, in light of the REMIS results, it regulated this supposed therapy.

Philip Noguchi, an FDA official who oversees cell therapies, said that as an experimental treatment lymphocyte immune therapy should have FDA approval, but that it had never been sought or granted. Indeed he allowed that the FDA did not know about the widespread use of this treatment until I had raised the question. "Appropriate action is being initiated," Noguchi said.

On January 30, 2002, the FDA sent a letter to Beer and others who still offered lymphocyte immune therapy. The letter informed them that they would have to receive permission from the agency to test this "investigational new drug." Beer later told me that Finch University would not support his investigational new drug application, so he resigned his position there. In late 2003, the Alan E. Beer Center for Reproductive Immunology & Genetics operated satellite clinics in Chicago, London, and Los Gatos, California.

In October 2003, I visited a bulletin board on the Yahoo Web site that attracted many of Beer's patients. This cybersalon, where patients swapped their tales of loss and triumph, included extensive discussions about lymphocyte immune therapy, which people in the United States now traveled to Mexico to receive.

· · ·

By the time the REMIS study ended, abundant evidence challenged the mechanisms that Beer proposed. Likewise, Medawar's idea about the fetus as a foreign graft seemed more wobbly than ever. As Carole Ober stressed to me, "there is no evidence that the mother's immune system reacts in a negative way against fetal cells."

Ober came to head the REMIS study because she had done fundamental genetic studies on miscarriage and immunity in the Hutterites of South Dakota. An Anabaptist sect of pacifist farmers, the Hutterites originated in the Tyrolean Alps in 1528, migrated to Russia, and in the 1870s again moved en masse, this time to the United States. About four hundred Hutterites formed communal farms, or colonies, in what is now the state of South Dakota. Ober in 1982 began genetic studies of the Schmiedeleut Hutterite colonies in South Dakota, a group that descended from sixty-four ancestors. These highly inbred, highly fertile Hutterites, who at the time produced an average of nine children per family, provided an excellent population in which Ober and her coworkers could examine some of the leading theories about immunology and pregnancy.

The cellular bar codes that allow the immune system to detect self from nonself contain a family of proteins known as human leukocyte antigens, or HLAs. Scientists to date have discovered nine different genes that produce these proteins. Each gene (referred to as HLA-A, HLA-B, etc.) comes in dozens of variations, and together they create a system that allows each person to have a unique bar code. In 1986, Ober began to follow Hutterite couples—who, on average, genetically resemble first cousins once removed—and their attempts to have children.

Beer's main miscarriage thesis hinges on the idea that a mother must recognize a fetus as foreign, which prods her immune system to produce blocking antibodies that stop other immune cells from attacking the invader. When couples have too much HLA similarity, he contends, the mother does not produce the blocking antibodies, leaving the fetus vulnerable to attack. As he put it to me, "compatibility breeds autoimmune contempt."

Ober tracked more than 250 pregnancies in 111 Hutterite couples. Nearly 85 percent made it to term. After studying the group for twelve years and following the reproductive history of some five hundred married women, Ober's group did not find one case of a woman who had three consecutive miscarriages, and all the women who had had three or more miscarriages gave birth to at least two live children. "It's not clear whether what we're seeing in the Hutterites has any bearing on recurrent miscarriage," Ober told me.

The Hutterite study did find that the couples with the closest HLA matches had the most miscarriages. But even in these cases, Ober saw no indication of immune rejection. Rather, she suspected that these couples shared an HLA gene, or some other gene that traveled with it, that directly had a negative effect on pregnancy. (In other mammals, studies have shown that HLA-like genes can affect embryo and fetal development.) "We have couples that are nearly identical to each other with regard to HLA—they are as close as sisters and brothers—and even though they have an increased miscarriage rate, they have lots of kids," Ober said.

The HLA story took another odd turn with the discovery in 1986 of a novel HLA molecule in trophoblasts, the critical cells that invade the uterine wall and later form the placenta. Trophoblasts create the interface between mother and baby, the place where they actually touch each other, so they are a logical place to start the attack if the maternal immune system regards the newcomer as a foreigner. Unlike other HLAs, this novel molecule found on trophoblasts, called HLA-G, differs remarkably little from person to person. As a result, the parts of the placenta that work most closely with the mother do not appear foreign.

HLA-G suggests that, contrary to Medawar, the placenta does not look like a transplanted organ or skin graft. Yet scientists have not dismissed the idea that a mother's immune system must somehow tolerate a baby: a fetus is genetically distinct from its mother, and the fetus and mother traffic cells between each other. Many scientists believe the immune interaction with the embryo has an entirely different mechanism from the one Medawar and his followers imagined. And in this rewriting of the orthodoxy, HLA-G occupies center stage.

Many researchers now believe that the maternal immune system can lead to a miscarriage by dispatching so-called natural killer cells to attack trophoblasts. But natural killer cells do not have the sophisticated ability to recognize the fine genetic differences between a mother and her embryo's cells. Rather, these primitive warriors have a cruder system that destroys any trophoblast if it completely lacks HLA molecules on its surface. The presence of HLA-G thus prevents attack by natural killer cells, and, because the molecule does not appear foreign, the trophoblast remains undetected by the more refined immune soldiers.

Clinical results bolster HLA-G's importance. Ober, Stephenson, Scott, and other REMIS investigators analyzed HLA-G in 113 couples who participated in the landmark recurrent miscarriage study. The researchers discovered two mutations in the HLA-G gene that increased the risk of miscarriage, an indication that a malfunctioning HLA-G could lead to a loss. A research group in Germany similarly linked HLA-G mutations to recurrent miscarriage. Yet another study with in vitro fertilization patients found that pregnancy occurred only with embryos that made measurable levels of the form of HLA-G that courses through a mother's bloodstream.

Contradictory results challenge many of these findings, which in 2001 led prominent, pioneering scientists in the field to publish a paper together titled "HLA-G Remains a Mystery." But HLA-G also represents the edge of knowledge today. It may solve the riddle of how a woman's immune system makes peace with the genetically foreign baby growing inside of her, and lead to therapies that make peace when a pregnant woman's immune system wages unnecessary war.

Medical experts continue to criticize clinicians who promote new, experimental immune therapies to prevent miscarriages for which enthusiasm outstrips evidence that they work. In September 2003 Michael Weisman, the director of the division of rheumatology at Cedars-Sinai Medical Center in Los Angeles, and his colleague Daniel Wallace took such a stand in a Journal of Rheumatology editorial. They told the story of a thirty-seven-year-old corporate attorney who had come to their center after four failed in vitro fertilizations. Referred to their center because she had "prevailed upon her gynecologist" to prescribe yet another experimental immune intervention popularized by Alan Beer, her case had given Weisman and Wallace great pause. In addition to aspirin and heparin, the woman wanted to take a drug that supposedly offsets the damage caused by natural killer cells.

The drug inhibits tumor necrosis factor-alpha, or TNF-α, a biochemical secreted by natural killer cells. TNF-α belongs to a family of immune system messengers that turn on or off production of antibodies and other immune troops. In the mid-1980s, researchers made the astonishing discovery that these messengers divided into two groups, dubbed Th1 and Th2, that cross-regulate each other in a seesaw fashion: high levels of Th1 mean low levels of Th2, and vice versa. TNF-α belongs to the Th1 group. When immunologists find an abundance of it, they can hear the creak of the spigot shutting off Th2 immunity.

Th1 messengers crank up the cellular machinery that sends out the immune system's Green Berets, the sharpshooters that can distinguish, say, a healthy cell from one that harbors a virus. These Green Berets can then destroy that cell. Th2 messengers crank up production of antibodies, which latch onto foreigners before they can infect cells. Several research groups have contended that a healthy pregnancy creates a Th2 immune state, theoretically by increasing levels of antibodies that prevent natural killer cells from harming the trophoblasts that go on to form the placenta. This hugely controversial hypothesis conversely suggests that Th1 messengers, like TNF-α, predominate in women who have recurrent miscarriages.

The FDA by then had approved three different drugs that inhibit TNF-α, primarily to treat rheumatoid arthritis. The regulations allow doctors to prescribe a licensed drug for any reason, a practice known as "off-label" use. Beer and others had begun prescribing these TNF-α inhibitors to miscarriage patients, like the woman described in the *Journal of Rheumatology* editorial.

As the editorial explained, after this woman began the treatment, she became pregnant and subsequently gave birth to a healthy five-pound, seven-ounce boy the next February. Weisman and Wallace noted that it was "impossible to know" whether the TNF-α inhibitor she took helped her carry to term, and they strongly questioned the safety of these drugs in pregnant women, as well as the rationale behind their use.

The drugs—Enbrel, Remicade, and Humira—"very likely could have profound effects upon the immune system that might present special pregnancy concerns, such as susceptibility to specific infections or unwanted influences upon development of the fetal immune system," they warned. Weisman and Wallace also lambasted the very idea of "reproductive immunologists" even prescribing immune therapies that remain "controversial at best." Disgusted, they wrote, "As far as we are able to determine, there are no recognized standards or board certifications that must be met or obtained for a physician to call him/herself a reproductive immunologist."

Beer and other ob-gyns who prescribed the drugs to miscarriage patients obviously believed the potential benefits outweighed the risks. Indeed, Beer prescribed Enbrel to his own daughter, Margaret Lindsey.

A nurse at San Francisco General Hospital, Lindsey, then thirty-four, had deep respect and admiration for her father, who had helped her and her husband through a most difficult chapter in their lives. In June 1999, Lindsey, seven weeks pregnant with what would be her second child, went to Chicago to visit her parents. "Being my father, he of course said, 'Let's just do an ultrasound and make sure everything's OK,'" she said. "It didn't look good."

An abnormal ultrasound prompted Beer to commission extensive blood work, and, when it was clear that she was about to miscarry, he took a biopsy sample of the lining of her uterus, which showed high levels of natural killer cells. Her blood tests also indicated overly abundant levels of TNF-α. In all, Beer found that his daughter met the criteria for four of the five categories of immune problems that he had linked to miscarriages. "That was a really big pill to swallow," she told me. "Here I was his daughter, all my life I'd seen him doing this stuff, and I'm thinking, there's just no way. The irony was too much."

Among other treatments she tried after this miscarriage, Lindsey did lymphocyte immune therapy and took the TNF-α inhibitor Enbrel. In February 2001, she became pregnant with twins, but only one had a heart and the pregnancy was not viable. Not only had their difficulties begun to weigh on Lindsey and her husband, it also took a toll on her father. "This was an emotionally wrenching time for him," she said.

By August, Lindsey had tallied three more miscarriages. "I was just sick and tired of the whole thing," she said. "It's sucking the life out of you. It's emotionally draining. I miscarried that month. Just another short one. I said I'm done. I'm really done. Gave away all my baby stuff."

Like many women who have a child and then repeatedly miscarry, Lindsey seriously inventoried her life. "I thought, you know, I've got a beautiful family, this is going to be fine," she concluded. Still, it nagged at her that she and her husband both came from large families, and she did not want her son to grow up an only child. Adoption did not interest them, but maybe they should have a go with IVF? In the end, her resolute decision melted away, and she opted for another round with her father. She became pregnant the first month. Give it a couple of weeks and it will be over, she thought. "But that pregnancy just did not quit."

Six months later, Lindsey felt odd and asked her father to check her blood. Spikes of natural killer cells and TNF-α prompted him to prescribe another round of lymphocyte immune therapy. Her levels returned to normal within a week. "Had I not done it, I'm convinced I would have lost the pregnancy," she told me. On May 7, 2002, Margaret Lindsey gave birth to a daughter and named her Alaina, after her grandfather.

The next day, Alan Beer asked his daughter whether she wanted to try for another child. "Dad, I just can't."

"Thank God," said Beer.

Lindsey laughed. "He would have, but he was relieved not to."

We reviewed the attacks on her father's work, which she well knew. "No matter what he did, or what anyone does who is on cutting edge, there's always going to be criticism," she said. "He's a very focused, driven man. He's so completely sincere and so concerned about each one of these people." And like many of Beer's patients, Lindsey had no doubt that his care helped her birth a child. "Scientists are going to argue it very differently than I would," she said. "It's going to always go on. It's going to go on until the day he dies. He's determined this is a science. It's not witchcraft. It's very specific medicine that's very complicated."

I recounted for her the results from the old Norwegian study about the power of tender-loving care alone. "I can tell you he does provide a lot of that," she said.

I do not presume to judge whether Alan Beer's treatment of his daughter led to the birth of his granddaughter Alaina. I do think that the aggressive interventions that he advocated for his own daughter add an interesting layer of complexity to the man. A doctor who gives the same treatment to his own child powerfully attests to his sincerity and conviction, which, to women who desperately want to carry a baby to term, often speak much louder than scientific evidence. I suspect that he does offer tender-loving care, and that its benefits may confuse the results his patients experience with experimental treatments. And I fully agree with Margaret Lindsey that the controversies will rage for years to come. Test-tube experiments and clinical studies, even rigorous ones, will never displace the ambiguity surrounding immune interventions as long as treated women continue to deliver healthy babies and suffer no obvious harm themselves. And the faith that couples have in treatments, as dubious as they may seem, on occasion will pay off.

When my friend Jess gave birth to her daughter in August 1999, she knew nothing of the negative findings from the REMIS study, and she assumed that lymphocyte immune therapy played a critical role in her successful outcome.

Scant evidence suggested that Jess had an immune problem that warranted injections with her husband's white blood cells, and yet given her past problems and her unequivocal success following the treatment, she understandably found it attractive to think that one led to the other. But I think the REMIS findings, the best study of lymphocyte immune therapy, make a compelling case that the therapy did not help any of those women. If anything, the results indicate that the treatment lowered their chances of carrying to term.

A coda to Jess's story casts further doubts about the value of lymphocyte immune therapy and spotlights the pitfalls of anecdotes. In the summer of 2001, with no intervention whatsoever, Jess, to her astonishment, became pregnant. In April 2002, she once again gave birth to a healthy baby girl.

5

BLACK SWANS

SCIENCE OFTEN MOVES FORWARD BY SERENDIPITY, WITH the study of one problem leading to a finding that affects a seemingly unrelated one. At London's St. Mary's Hospital, the same place where Lesley Regan runs a recurrent miscarriage clinic and James Mowbray tested lymphocyte immunization, Alexander Fleming famously discovered penicillin because a spore traveled from the lab a floor below his own and contaminated one of his petri dishes. Researchers initially developed Viagra to treat heart disease and angina, but realized from side effects reported in early human studies that it could help men achieve and maintain an erection. Similarly, a confusing finding in patients with lupus led to the discovery of an immune reaction that clearly explains some miscarriages. And this advance should give pause to anyone who dismisses out of hand the assertion that as yet undefined errant immune responses cause pregnancy losses.

In lupus, the immune system fails to distinguish self from nonself and attacks its own tissue, causing skin rashes, swollen joints, and organ damage. In the early 1950s, lupus researchers stumbled across a conundrum in some of their patients, whose antibody tests for syphilis turned positive even though they did not have the disease. Other lupus patients paradoxically experienced blood clots despite the fact that their blood was rich with a "lupus anticoagulant" that supposedly *prevents* the thickening of blood. A 1954 paper did link this lupus anticoagulant to one woman's eight miscarriages. But nearly three decades passed before researchers uncovered the connections among antibodies to this anticoagulant, the syphilis antibody test, and pregnancy loss.

The breakthrough came in 1983 when Graham Hughes, head of the lupus unit at St. Thomas' Hospital in London, and his team developed a more precise test for these antibodies. Using this improved technique, they described a set of female patients who tested positive for both the syphilis antibody and the lupus anticoagulant. These lupus patients had "sticky blood," triggered by a collection of antibodies now known to be responsible for "antiphospholipid syndrome." They also had a high rate of miscarriages, which later research suggests occurred because these antibodies affect both implantation and blood clotting.

E. Nigel Harris, a rheumatologist then working under Hughes, said colleagues, wary of immune-based explanations of miscarriage, at first expressed great skepticism when they presented their finding at meetings. "I almost felt like persona non grata," said Harris, now dean of the Morehouse School of Medicine in Atlanta, Georgia. At one meeting, however, an elderly physician spoke up not to attack him, but to explain why the idea met so much resistance. The man believed their findings, but said that linking antibodies to fetal loss reminded him of the black swan: the rare bird exists, but it sounds fictional. Harris and a colleague started calling the antiphospholipid antibody–miscarriage connection the "Syndrome of the Black Swan." And "For obvious reasons, we decided that the initials B.S. should not be used in referring to the syndrome," he later joked in one of his many papers about their discovery.

At eighteen, Rani McAuley thought she did not want children. Rani, now twenty-six, told me about this decision, rolling her eyes and shaking her head. Four years later, she and her husband, John, who live in East London, thrilled to the birth of their baby boy.

Eight weeks after giving birth, Rani dozed off with her son sleeping on her lap. When her sister walked in the room, an odd detail marred the typically serene scene of an exhausted new mother napping with her newborn: the baby had stopped breathing. Rani's sister resuscitated the infant, and they called an ambulance. At the hospital, doctors put him on a ventilator, but the brain damage had taken its toll, and he died. "I felt so guilty," said Rani. She knew she had done nothing wrong, that he had died from what the English call "cot death" and Americans refer to as "sudden infant death syndrome." But still.

Seven months later, Rani, as the British say, "fell pregnant," but, a few weeks later, she miscarried. Four months later, Rani was pregnant again. At twelve weeks, she had an ultrasound. "I was petrified," Rani said. But everything looked fine, and at the three-month milestone she relaxed. "I thought I was past the danger zone." A few weeks later, cramping and a vaginal discharge heralded a possible miscarriage. At the hospital, an ultrasound indicated that all was well. But that night, her water broke, and she lost the child. Another four months passed, and in the winter of 2002, Rani became pregnant yet again. This time, she miscarried before the sixth week. "The first baby I carried, that's what gave me hope," said Rani. "But I thought there was something seriously wrong, and I thought I'd never be able to have a baby."

Rani's ob-gyn referred her to the Recurrent Miscarriage Clinic at London's St. Mary's Hospital. The doctors assessed her fallopian tubes and uterus, but it was the blood tests they did that revealed her underlying problem: she had antiphospholipid syndrome.

Given this finding, when Rani became pregnant again in the winter of 2003, she followed the recommendations of the doctors at St. Mary's, who prescribed daily doses of baby aspirin and injections of heparin (a complex sugar made by the body that prevents blood clotting), a treatment that this clinic had helped pioneer. "I feel good about this, but I do get scared at night," Rani told me when, halfway through the problem-free pregnancy, I met her and her husband, John, at a St. Mary's checkup. "If anything went wrong this time, I don't know what I'd do. People hear about miscarriage, and they don't take it seriously. I never did before. People don't realize."

"It shows you how fragile life is," added John.

On December 7, 2003, Rani gave birth to a healthy baby girl. When I spoke with her one month later, she said, "We're over the moon, happy."

· · ·

Antiphospholipid syndrome remains controversial, so much so that one research group in a 2002 paper called it the "immunological Wars of the Roses." But the hottest debates now have less to do with whether these antibodies cause miscarriages than they do with determining the stage of pregnancy at which they cause problems, what they specifically disrupt, and how best to subdue them.

At first, many investigators thought antiphospholipid syndrome mainly caused second-trimester miscarriages through sticky blood forming clots in the placenta. Supporting this idea, treatment with aspirin and heparin, both of which thin the blood, appeared to work in women who had a history of late losses. But in 1996 William Kutteh, a recurrent miscarriage specialist then at the University of Texas Southwestern Medical Center in Dallas, published a study that showed how aspirin and heparin also could prevent first-trimester miscarriages. The next year, Lesley Regan's group at St. Mary's published still more convincing evidence that this treatment helped prevent first-trimester loss.

At the St. Mary's recurrent miscarriage clinic, which conducted the world's largest study to assess the frequency of this problem, researchers found elevated levels of antiphospholipid antibodies in 15 percent of five hundred women who each had three or more consecutive losses. In these women, the researchers discovered that 90 percent who became pregnant again would miscarry without treatment. As Regan, Raj Rai, and their coworkers documented in the British Medical Journal in 1997, they looked at ninety of these women, who had had an average of four previous miscarriages (one had fifteen), the majority in the first trimester. Of the forty-five women who received aspirin alone, just over 40 percent carried to term. The forty-five women who also took heparin had a success rate of just over 70 percent. All but four of the thirty-nine miscarriages in the study occurred during the first trimester. An editorial that accompanied the paper called these new interventions "a medical achievement worth celebrating."

Heparin has a few serious drawbacks: women must inject it, and its use can cause bone loss. This intervention also will not help most women. The British Medical Journal editorial acknowledged this limitation, but still emphasized that "the annual incidence of pregnancy loss among women in Britain alone because of this potentially treatable condition must be huge."

The careful design of this study persuaded many colleagues that an-tiphospholipid syndrome caused first-trimester miscarriages—as did Regan's reputation. She began her research career believing that wayward immune responses frequently cause fetal loss. But after a time in the field, she switched sides, becoming a self-described "debunker." She told me she thought Medawar's hypothesis of the fetal graft was more noise than signal. "I think it stopped progress," she said. "An enormous amount of time has been spent in explaining or trying to find data to substantiate this hypothesis." She singled out Alan Beer's Web site for offering a "mountain of information" that had never been published in a high-qual-ity, peer-reviewed journal. "I'm absolutely amazed at how gullible people are when they read these reports," she said. Yet antiphospholipid anti-bodies had convinced Regan that maternal antibodies could, in this se-lect case, lead to many miscarriages.

Regan's group in 2002 published a stunning study that questioned the prevailing wisdom about how antiphospholipids caused first-trimester miscarriages. The researchers rejected the theory that sticky blood led to blood clots in the placenta, instead arguing that the anti-bodies primarily interfered with the process of implantation.

In this study, they examined 135 "products of conception" from the first trimester: 31 specimens exhibited normal karyotypes and came from women who had antiphospholipid syndrome, 50 with normal karyotypes came from women who did not have the syndrome, 34 had abnormal numbers of chromosomes, and another 20 came from women who elected to have abortions. They found no evidence of placental blood clots in any group.

The antiphospholipid antibodies, it appears, prevent the placental tro-phoblast cells from properly attaching to the mother's uterus. In women with the syndrome, about one in four had normal trophoblast invasion. Miscarriages from women who did not have the syndrome appeared to invade normally more than half the time, and, in elective abortions, proper attachment occurred in roughly three out of four instances.

Regan and her colleagues suggested that the antiphospholipid antibodies might disrupt trophoblast invasion either by binding to the tro-phoblasts or the maternal cells. Raj Rai, an ob-gyn who helps Regan run the miscarriage clinic, offered another possible explanation for these early losses: although heparin traditionally is thought of as a blood-thin-ning agent, it also can modulate immune responses. Blood clots, he pointed out, do not present much of a threat to an embryo or early fetus, which does not want much blood. And heparin seems to have an effect only during the first twelve weeks, adding to the supposition that it can-not work by preventing clots.

The spirited, even contentious, debates in the pages of scientific jour-nals that surround these ideas—and the worth of heparin and aspirin in preventing miscarriage—promise to roil the field for years to come. Yet today, other than the Rh factor, antiphospholipid syndrome has become what many investigators consider the most convincing case that an out-of-whack immune response can cause miscarriages. And the success with aspirin and heparin has led clinicians to test this treatment in pregnant women who have a variety of inherited blood-clotting problems.

After five years of marriage, Penny and Simon in 1994 decided to try and have a baby, and one month later, in September, Penny became pregnant. "It all seemed so easy," said Penny, a secretary in London with a sweet disposition and an open face that hides few emotions. She waited until she reached ten weeks before sharing the good news, and two weeks later, she went in for her first ultrasound. The fetus apparently had died a week earlier.

Penny became pregnant again in spring. This time, her first scan came at week thirteen. "We had prayed it would be OK this time as I had gone past the twelve-weeks milestone," she said. But again, the baby had died, and a potentially joyous doctor's visit turned into a heartbreaking day. Simon repeatedly assured his wife that they should not blame them-selves for the miscarriages. "Simon was brilliant, so supportive and kind," she said.

Three months later, for the third time within one year, Penny became pregnant. This time, at her insistence, Penny received an early scan at seven weeks. The woman performing the scan excused herself to go find a doctor. "We both knew what this meant," remembered Penny. "I had to return to the waiting room, amongst happily pregnant women, until the doctor could see me and tell me what I feared. It was just awful. I couldn't believe it was happening again."

Actually, it was even worse than she originally feared: Penny had a molar pregnancy, a rare and potentially dangerous situation in which an egg receives forty-six chromosomes from the father—sometimes without any from the mother—and then creates a placenta that often grows uncontrollably. Even after a dilation and curettage, tissue from molar pregnancies sometimes continues to grow, so doctors closely monitor the woman's human chorionic gonadotropin for several months and advise her not to become pregnant until those levels return to normal.

For Penny this took a year and a half. "People at work stopped asking me whether I was going to try again and looked at me with pity," she said. "I felt like a freak. I hated seeing babies and children everywhere I went, on the Tube, in the supermarket, just walking down the street. I even hated seeing advertisements with babies in them. My eyes would just fill up with tears and I would feel so miserable and pathetic. I am sure I was very difficult to live with, and how my marriage stayed afloat is down to the love and patience of my husband and family."

Penny's doctors at London's Royal Free Hospital could not find any explanation for her reproductive nightmare, and referred her to St. Mary's Recurrent Miscarriage Clinic. In the middle of testing at St. Mary's, Penny learned that her hCG levels had returned to normal. "I was so desperate for a baby by this stage that we tried again immediately," she said. Five weeks into her fourth pregnancy, she bled heavily, losing so much blood that she required an emergency transfusion.

Frustrated and angry, Penny concluded that she and Simon should abandon their dream. "That was it," she said. "I was never going to put myself or him in this untenable situation again, and he reluctantly agreed that I was probably right," she said. "Once out of the hospital, I refused to talk about it, and we went on like that for some months, just avoiding the subject but hurting all the time."

During those months, St. Mary's contacted Penny with her blood results. She had tested positive for factor V Leiden, the most common of at least nine inherited blood-clotting problems that researchers have implicated as a cause of miscarriage. No miscarriage intervention existed, they said, other than the tender-loving care that the clinic would offer her.

In January 1998, doctors diagnosed Simon's mother with leukemia, predicting that she would live less than four years. "This news acted like a wake-up call for me," Penny said. "I realized that I was being selfish in not persevering with my goal to have a baby and give her a grandchild." Terrified, Penny and Simon restarted their pregnancy quest. She became pregnant within three months, and, at seven weeks, nervously went in to St. Mary's for an ultrasound, staring at the ceiling as the doctor scanned her uterus. Then she heard the words she had only imagined. "Look, there's the heartbeat," the doctor said. In January 1999, she gave birth to a daughter, Lily. "When Lily was born, I felt fulfilled and the happiest I have ever known," she said.

Three years passed, and Penny told Simon she wanted to try to have a second child. Why push our luck? he asked. But Penny persisted and in July 2002 scored yet another positive pregnancy test. When she went to St. Mary's, she learned that new research suggested that it made sense to treat pregnant women with factor V Leiden with aspirin and heparin, the same intervention used for antiphospholipid syndrome.

Although no rigorous clinical trial had proven that the intervention would work for women with factor V Leiden, the clinic recently had studied a small group of pregnant women with the inherited disorder who had miscarried early at least three times, did not have antiphospholipid syndrome, and had not attempted any intervention. Nearly two-thirds miscarried, while in a larger group of similar women who did not have the disorder, only one-third had a pregnancy loss. This difference, combined with a few small studies that suggested the benefits of aspirin and heparin, tipped the scales in favor of treatment. Penny did it, and sailed through the pregnancy, giving birth to their second daughter, Lydia, in April 2003. "There was a time when I nearly gave up all hope, but my experience has taught me to tell others to keep going and, at the same time, not to allow it to rule their lives, even when they feel the darkest despair," she said.

Penny's story holds another lesson. Clearly, she did not *need* heparin and aspirin to carry a baby to term, as Lily's birth proved. But if the treatment indeed makes a difference for women who have factor V Leiden and other clotting disorders, they increase their odds of success—which is the most that any miscarriage interventions can promise.

The tests that identify antiphospholipid syndrome, factor V Leiden, and other blood-clotting problems share this shortcoming: They rely on the presence of antibodies or proteins associated with the condition, not on evidence of clotting abnormalities. To steer around this obstacle, Raj Rai of St. Mary's turned to thromboelastography, a half-century-old test that measures the elasticity of blood.

Originally described in 1948, thromboelastography measures the rate at which blood clots. It accomplishes this tricky feat with a machine outfitted with a small cup that rotates a blood sample from side to side, gauging the strength of clots. In December 2003, Rai and his coworkers published the first evidence that the test can help identify clotting problems in women who have had at least three consecutive miscarriages. The study examined the blood of 494 such women who had no known underlying problem and an age-matched group of 55 women with no history of miscarriages. The blood of the women with multiple miscarriages contained significantly stronger blood clots than that of the women who had not miscarried. What's more, looking at the recurrent miscarriage group alone, the women who had stronger clots had a much higher risk of a loss if they became pregnant again.

In 2004, Rai and colleagues had a trial under way to test whether two baby aspirins a day can more effectively reduce clot strength than a single dose, and whether this prescription, in turn, reduces the miscarriage rate.

Fifteen years ago, when Sue Cocke was twenty-five, she stopped having periods. Cocke and her husband, convinced that they could not have children, arranged to adopt a baby from a thirteen-year-old girl. Cocke, a nurse who then lived in Kentucky, attended the delivery. But then the birth mom's family persuaded her to renege on the deal. Cocke and her husband went home empty-handed. "We decided we'll have one of our own, and no one will take it away."

Cocke tried Clomid, which coaxes the body into ovulating, but it failed. Next, she injected another ovulation stimulant, Pergonal (menotropins), and at twenty-seven, became pregnant but quickly miscarried. "I was squashed, but I got pregnant, which meant I could do it again," said Cocke. A few months later, she tested pregnant and miscarried the same day.

The next year, Cocke became pregnant for the third time. In her twenty-eighth week, an ugly pain in her legs sent her to the hospital. This bout with leg pain was not her first. A couple of years earlier, a similar jolt landed her in an emergency room. This time a doctor diagnosed a pulled muscle. "So I slept Sunday night in the bathtub because it hurt to have the sheet on my leg," she said. "I kept saying I think I have a clot."

They found a clot, and dosed her with heparin. The next week, during a doctor's appointment, she had trouble seeing straight. Her blood pressure tested so high that the doctor told her "you just bought a ticket to the hospital." Blood work revealed elevated levels of antiphospholipid antibodies. As luck would have it, E. Nigel Harris, the developer of the powerful new test for these miscarriage-linked antibodies, had just joined the medical team treating her.

Cocke had preeclampsia, a life-threatening high blood pressure for both mother and baby that typically begins during the second trimester. Although investigators have pointed to many suspected causes—including antiphospholipid antibodies—the only known effective cure is giving birth. Cocke's blood pressure rose so high that the doctors said they might have to perform a cesarean section, a terrible prospect because her clotting problem ruled out anesthesia. But then her blood pressure inexplicably turned around and the hospital staff sent her home. Cocke immediately returned a maternity dress that she had yet to wear. "I wasn't going to do this again," she said.

The next Saturday, while making lasagna, Cocke "just didn't feel right." She returned to the hospital, and on Sunday, it hurt to focus her eyes. "When my husband came to visit, I said, 'Don't talk to me and don't ask me to talk to you,'" recalled Cocke, who had to sit in a "cardiac chair" to relieve her screaming high blood pressure. "I remember my husband said to the doctor, 'When I left her she was bad. She's worse. What's going on?'"

The next day, Cocke felt what she thought was her baby's first kick. Later she realized that the pain was the placenta breaking off the uterine wall. Then came the worst news an expectant mother can hear. "They looked at me and said, 'There's no heartbeat, your baby has died,'" she said. "And they left me." When her husband arrived, she told him the baby had died. Then her doctor walked in and informed them that she, too, was in grave danger. "If we don't do something soon we're going to lose her, too," he said.

"I kept making deals with God," recalled Cocke, who hoped that the fetal monitor was simply wrong.

On Tuesday morning, they wheeled her to labor and delivery. "The nurse put on a monitor, but only one—for my contractions, not the fetal heartbeat," she said. "It's like, Don't say it so it won't be real. Then they came in and said, 'Do you smoke or drink?' I said, 'No, but I will. What do you have?'"

After Cocke repeatedly complained that she had to go to the bathroom, two nurses and a resident helped her to the toilet. Inside the bowl, they placed a stainless-steel "hat" to catch whatever came out. "I delivered right there, into the hat," she said. It was 7:20 A.M. on May 24, 1988. The baby boy was two pounds, nine ounces, and eighteen inches long, with blond curls. They named him Edward Fitzgerald.

When she left the bathroom, she asked to see her son. "In one of the most poignant moments of my life, they put him on my chest," she said. "My heart was beating so fast I thought it would jump-start his heart. And his jaw fell open. At that moment, I would have traded everything to have heard him take one breath."

On the drive home from the hospital, Sue Cocke noticed kids not wearing their seat belts in another car. "You just want to go up to them and scream, 'Do you know how fast they'll be gone?'" She also soon recognized that she had hardened, in a way that stunned her. "You almost get callous about things. 'What can you do to me at this point? There's nothing you can do to me.'"

A few months later, she went to see E. Nigel Harris.

"What do you do all day?" he asked.

"I sit around and cry," she said.

"I would, too," he replied.

"Right then I loved him," Sue told me.

She quickly became pregnant again, and at twenty-two weeks started spotting. She went in for an ultrasound. When the technician said, "Let me go get the doctor," Sue started to cry. She knew.

In the spring of 1989, Cocke became pregnant again. An ultrasound showed nothing, and they asked her to come back the next week.

On the next ultrasound, a heartbeat appeared. "I'll be damned," said Sue.

E. Nigel Harris knew of reports from a few groups that successfully treated recurrent miscarriage by injecting women with antibodies pooled from several people. So-called intravenous immunoglobulin, or IVIG, had never proven itself in a randomized, controlled clinical trial, but maybe, by some as yet unproven mechanism, pooled antibodies could counteract the deleterious effects of the antiphospholipid antibodies. It was fighting with fire. Cocke agreed to the injections.

Unlike lymphocyte immune therapy, IVIG by then had received approval from the Food and Drug Administration. First licensed in 1981 to treat antibody-deficient people, it subsequently also won the FDA's blessing to treat other relatively rare immune disorders. Harris and others, taking advantage of the off-label use regulations that allow doctors to prescribe an approved drug as they see fit, began offering IVIG to some miscarriage patients. Cocke's main concern was the steep cost of what the doctors called this "liquid gold." Harris assured her that the hospital would cover the expense of repeated IVIG infusions, which can run as high as $20,000.

On January 15, 1990, Sue Cocke, twenty-eight weeks pregnant, noticed a slowdown in her baby's movements. The doctors and nurses monitored her closely, and when they lost the baby's heartbeat, they performed an emergency cesarean.

She had given birth to a perfectly healthy three-pound, fifteen-ounce son, whom they named William. "It's the hardest thing I've ever had to do," she told me, "and it's the best thing I've ever done."

Sue Cocke attributes William's birth to her IVIG treatment. But whether IVIG had anything to do with William's birth remains speculation. Six small-scale, randomized, controlled trials in the 1990s evaluated its ability to prevent miscarriage, but they had different outcomes, and none had enough patients to come up with definitive results. In 2000, Mary Stephenson launched a four-year, 180-women study in hopes of assessing IVIG's worth.

Several research groups have proposed mechanisms to explain how IVIG might help avert a miscarriage. Some experiments show that IVIG suppresses natural killer cells, which appear to disrupt implantation. Indeed, studies suggest that women who repeatedly miscarry chromosomally normal babies produce higher levels of natural killer cells. Others contend that IVIG speeds up the rate at which the body breaks down antiphospholipid antibodies. To date, no clear-cut mechanism has surfaced.

Maybe IVIG is another black swan. Experimental medicines, however, are not innocent until proven guilty; rather, they remain suspect until proven worthwhile, as all have the potential of causing harm. IVIG inadvertently infected people with hepatitis C: contaminations occurred both before and after 1989, the year scientists first isolated the virus that causes the disease. Although revised regulatory standards minimize the risk of contamination, no amount of screening can test for a pathogen that science has yet to discover.

I do not mean to imply that the risk of IVIG outweighs its benefits. But for desperate couples experiencing repeated miscarriages, untried options can have an intoxicating effect, leading them to throw caution to the wind. Confusing matters further still, women often pile IVIG on top of so many other interventions that it becomes impossible to judge which therapy deserves credit. Sometimes, women have more than one underlying medical condition creating their problem. Maybe these treatments help, maybe not. But this much I know for certain: women who have had several miscarriages and then carry to term after intervening with immune treatments will, by and large, ascribe their success to whatever they took.

Even experienced bird watchers get carried away by enthusiasm when they think they have seen a rare bird. Report a Chihuahuan raven sighting in Vermont, and dozens of seasoned birders will race to the site and claim to have seen the creature, only to have someone capture a close-up photograph that clearly shows the squared-off tail of a crow. The same holds true for the black swans in medicine: claims of sightings, when closely scrutinized, most often fall apart.

E. Nigel Harris explicitly addressed this phenomenon in the closing of "Syndrome of the Black Swan," his editorial about antiphospholipid syndrome. "A word of warning," wrote Harris. "Although patients with the antiphospholipid syndrome exist, they (like black swans) are probably not found as frequently as enthusiastic medical personnel might like. Only a small fraction of all patients with thrombosis or fetal loss will have this syndrome, but the numbers are large enough and complications severe enough to justify searching for them."

6

THE CYCLE OF LIFE

WAY BACK IN THE FOURTH CENTURY B.C., ARISTOTLE CON-tended that life began in menstrual blood. The blood mixed with semen, he thought, to form an embryo. A millennium later, Saint Isidore of Seville promoted an equally misguided perception about menses: "On contact with this gore, crops do not generate, wine goes sour, trees lose their fruit, iron is corrupted by rust, copper is blackened. Should dogs eat any of it they go mad."

Colin Finn, a veterinary surgeon and implantation researcher based at the University of Liverpool's Veterinary Field Station, resurrects this history in a mind-stretching 1996 essay, "Why Do Women Menstruate?" It was not until the beginning of the twentieth century that scientists first began to puzzle together how hormones orchestrate the menstrual cycle, discovering, in the words of one gynecologist in 1910, that menstruation "was a secondary process, a degeneration of the mucous membrane which from a failure of pregnancy has not been able to fulfil [sic] its function." But the deeper, evolutionary question of why women bleed each month during their reproductive years remains unanswered. And explorations of this mystery and the roles that hormones play help to explain how the timing of the precisely regulated menstrual cycle plays an essential role in supporting—or undermining—a pregnancy.

Except for primates, few species menstruate. Finn and others argue that humans evolved this cyclical shedding of the uterine lining as a by-product of a defensive mechanism to protect mothers from their embryos.

When reptiles branched off from amphibians and started laying hard-shelled eggs on land, the embryo had to develop membranes to stay hydrated and to eliminate wastes. These evolved into the amnion, famous today because of the fetal chromosomal test that samples amniotic fluid, and the allantois, a precursor to the placenta. In the next huge leap, vertebrates began to carry their own offspring—the "viviparity" that Medawar wrote about—and different species established dramatically different mechanisms to allow the foreigner to grow inside the uterus.

Embryos from humans, other primates, and some rodents exhibit distinctly aggressive behavior toward their mothers, which Finn and others believe explains why women menstruate. Successful implantation occurs only if the embryo properly "invades" the lining of the uterus, which requires that the placenta's trophoblast cells penetrate deeply, boring into maternal arteries to shunt blood to the growing baby. If the mother did not stop the trophoblasts' drilling, they might burrow so deeply into her uterus that she could hemorrhage and die. So the uterus developed an ingenious strategy to allow invasion but then, by changing its cellular structure, stop the process. As the pathologist Harvey Kliman, head of Yale University's Reproductive and Placental Research Unit, explained it to me, the uterine lining "changes from soil into bricks."

But why do women menstruate cyclically, as opposed to just maintaining the soil until an embryo implants and then turning it to bricks? Finn explored this idea in depth in another, still grander essay he wrote a few years later. He dismissed a theory, popularized in the early 1990s, that menstruation evolved to clear the uterus of pathogens brought in by sperm, which made little sense, he contended, if only because most viviparous species do not menstruate. For similar reasons, he had little use for the idea that menstruation exists as a miscarriage mechanism, ridding the body of unimplanted embryos. He outright mocked the "imaginative" suggestion made in 1930 that menstruation "provides women with vicarious sexual satisfaction, thus preserving their virginity." And he also made a convincing counterargument to the hypothesis that it saved metabolic energy by only occasionally preparing the uterus for implantation. Indefinitely maintaining the uterine soil, Finn argued, would prevent the preimplantation state of the lining in which uterine glands secrete biochemicals that prepare sperm for fertilization and help transport them to the egg.

Curious about why humans and a few other species would have evolved invasive trophoblasts, in 2003 I e-mailed Finn, who by then had retired. His answer delighted me, more for its characteristic scientific restraint than for its insight. "What brought it about is anyone's guess (like most things in evolutionary biology)," he wrote back. "The easiest way is to put it down to chance random mutations, which over millions of years proved advantageous to the species. Unless you are religious, what more can one say?"

Regardless of how women came to have a cycle, because they do, timing is everything. Indeed, Finn in 1974 published one of the first papers to propose that a "window of implantation" exists. This idea received solid confirmation two decades later from the study led by Allen Wilcox, the North Carolina "King of Pee" who conducted the famous daily urine testing of 221 women for six months.

In addition to clarifying that the fertility window remains open for five days before ovulation and on the actual day, Wilcox and colleagues demonstrated from their urine samples that implantation works best between day 8 and day 10 after ovulation. During those few days—the middle of the "luteal phase" that stretches from ovulation to menses—the glands and stroma that make up the uterine lining become particularly velvety, an ideal place for an embryo to attach and then burrow. If the lining remains lush too long, the placenta will attach too deeply, with trophoblasts tunneling all the way through the uterus, leading to a potentially life-threatening situation for the mother. If the lining becomes inhospitable too early, as happens with what's called a deficient luteal phase, the embryo will not burrow, leading to a miscarriage, or it will not burrow properly, causing preeclampsia later in the pregnancy, a condition that causes dangerously high blood pressure in the mother.

Aristotle was wrong when he imagined menstrual blood as a primordial soup from which life springs. But he wasn't that wrong. Thanks to science, we now know the arrival of menses presages the body's readiness for conception and implantation, and that a cascade of hormones tightly regulate this process. But as much as medicine understands the biomechanics, when the cycle of life sputters and causes miscarriage, our ability to correct the problem has not advanced much beyond Aristotle's day.

"I never wanted children until I turned thirty-five," Marian Anderson, a television journalist who lives in Vancouver, told me. Anderson has the no-nonsense, fast-paced, wry demeanor that befits a reporter. "I never knew anything about the female reproduction cycle because it was of no interest to me," she said. But Anderson soon would become expert on such seemingly arcane topics as progesterone's relationship to luteinizing hormone, menopause and follicle-stimulating hormone, the uterine lining, and the ovulation window.

Her change of heart about rug rats occurred at thirty-five, when she started to bleed in the middle of her cycle. A visit to a gynecologist revealed fibroids—common, noncancerous tumors that grow in the uterus and might contribute to some miscarriages but typically go untreated. "If you want kids, start trying now," the gynecologist told her. At thirty-six, Anderson became pregnant. "It was the most unbelievable, simple pregnancy," she said. In March 1999, she gave birth to a healthy baby boy.

She conceived one year later, on her son's birthday, a coincidence of timing made more remarkable by the fact that she recognized and remembered it. "I just expected it to be easy again," she said. After a positive urine test at home, Anderson made a visit to her doctor, who, after failing to find a fetal heartbeat with a stethoscope, sent her to a technician for an ultrasound. "The woman doing the ultrasound insensitively kept saying, 'Why are you here? Are you sure you're pregnant? I don't see the child.'" Anderson had an empty gestational sac, a condition that occurs when the embryo fails to grow, which physicians commonly refer to as a "blighted" ovum (actually it is a blighted embryo). "I had never been that shocked," she said. "It was like being told you had cancer." That night, her husband of fifteen years had to work, and the emotional wallop hit her full force. "I just sat there alone and was hysterical, sobbing."

A few months later, in July 2000, Anderson tested positive again on a home urine stick, but then she quickly got her period. That September, she became pregnant for the third time since her son's birth. Eight weeks into the pregnancy, she had a transvaginal ultrasound, which can detect an embryo earlier than the familiar wand on the belly. Again, the technician detected a blighted ovum.

Anderson was referred to an obstetrician who had trained with Mary Stephenson, the head of Canada's largest recurrent miscarriage clinic. A thorough workup, which included blood tests and a sampling of the lining of her uterus—an "endometrial biopsy"—revealed two underlying problems. Anderson's blood tested highly positive for antiphospholipid antibodies. The endometrial biopsy suggested that she also had what's called a luteal phase deficiency, a controversial condition in which hormonal imbalances hamper implantation. Specifically, a dearth of progesterone leaves the uterine lining in a state that resembles a brick wall, rather than the fluffy, rich soil an embryo needs to implant. Anderson's clinician referred her to Stephenson, "the expert to see," said Anderson. But Stephenson, it turned out, had a six-month waiting list. "The clock's really ticking," said Anderson. "A six-month wait in a woman turning thirty-nine and freaking out."

Miscarriage exposes one's fragility, but less visibly, it also brings out a toughness, a sort of courage mixed with frustration and a dollop of rage. I asked her why she wanted a child so badly. "Someone said I couldn't," she said. "I also loved being a mommy. My whole new group—I went to Gymboree and Mother Goose—everyone had their second child and I didn't. I wanted to be a parent again."

Anderson threw herself at the subject, first studying antiphospholipid syndrome. "I combed every book and Internet site I could find," she said. "Several journals from scientific conferences. They were very hard for me to read. I read them forty-two times and underlined things in yellow. It seemed they consistently recommended the same treatment: start heparin the day after ovulation. And if Mary didn't agree, I'd be really angry. I came in with a briefcase full of research material. My husband thought she'd kick me out."

When Stephenson saw Anderson, she respectfully flipped through her collection of papers, making copies of a few of them. Stephenson confirmed Anderson's antiphospholipid syndrome, as well as a deficiency in her luteal phase. Just as Anderson had hoped, Stephenson prescribed daily heparin injections. Although Stephenson had serious reservations about the commonly used test to diagnose luteal phase deficiency, she also prescribed the most popular treatment for the problem, the hormone progesterone.

Given the success rate with heparin and the potential added benefit of progesterone, and hope being hope, Anderson lulled herself into believing that this time, everything would work fine. In May 2001, she became pregnant, but a heart did not beat on an early ultrasound. "That sunk me into a depression that was so great," Anderson said. "I could have been suicidal if I didn't already have a child."

Her depression intensified when she entered the hospital for a dilation and curettage in the same wing that women go to for abortions. "Everything on the wall had to do with abortion, birth control, and safe sex," Anderson remembered. "It was just awful. This was the most terrible experience of my life. I was completely and utterly mentally depressed." An analysis of tissue retrieved at the D and C showed no chromosomal abnormalities.

Anderson felt alone, isolated. "The first loss, I got flowers," she said. "The second, third, and fourth, I got nothing." Her supportive husband could not turn her depression around. "Men want to fix things," she said. "And they can't." Her friendships felt the strain, too. "No one—and I have lots of friends—gave me what I needed," she said. "To just say, 'Oh my God, that's terrible.' That's all I wanted someone to say." Making matters more complicated still, many of her closest women friends happened to be pregnant, and she shunned them. "I couldn't be around pregnant people," Anderson said. "I was around a girlfriend who was pregnant and complaining about having back pain. I could have hit her."

For three weeks after the miscarriage, Anderson slept little, trolling the Internet and her stack of fertility books for new ideas. She investigated adoption. "I could write books on fertility, miscarriage, and adoption based on what I know," she said. Naturopathic medicine particularly intrigued her. And she began to question the type of heparin she injected, as well as her progesterone dosage. "Miscarriage is so mysterious that it makes you feel completely out of control," she said. "I needed to feel like I was doing something to help myself."

Stephenson referred Anderson to a psychiatrist who specializes in "frequent loss." The psychiatrist recommended that she start antidepressants. "I said this is the issue: I don't want to be on any more drugs," she replied. "I just wanted someone to tell me, It's OK to be sad."

Anderson well recognized that she had become "absolutely obsessed." She began to monitor her cycle intensively, charting her temperature each day to find the rise that signaled ovulation and the start of the luteal phase. She spent several hundred dollars on a computerized ovulation predictor that charts the results of daily urine tests. For another indicator that one of her ovaries had released a ripe egg, she frequently checked her cervical mucus, which changes consistency at ovulation. After studying several books and papers about holistic methods of treating infertility and miscarriage, she started to take about forty vitamins and herb supplements a day, changed her diet, switched to a different heparin, and increased her progesterone. "Before having kids, I swore I'd never do this, and I thought people who are this obsessed and mechanical about conception are crazy," Anderson said. "But with what I'd gone through, if you told me to stand on one leg and recite the Gettysburg Address, I would have done it."

Long before the discovery of hormones, humans believed (based on the differences among castrated animals—and boys, for that matter) that the sex glands secreted special juices. From these insights came a subindustry of potions and elixirs manufactured from testicles and ovaries that had much more ambitious goals than preventing pregnancy loss.

Historians have dated the birth of endocrinology, the study of hormones, to May 31, 1889, when the renowned physiologist Charles-Édouard Brown-Séquard, then seventy-two, reported at the Société de Biologie in Paris that he had injected himself with extracts from dog and guinea pig testicles, which he claimed rejuvenated him. The loony rejuvenation theory, also called glandular therapy, became an international rage—tarnishing the idea of hormone-based treatment for decades. But Brown-Séquard accurately recognized a breathtaking medical opportunity. "There is, in short, a new therapeutics to create, in which the medicaments will be produced by the different tissues of the organism," he wrote in 1891, and the discovery three decades later that injections of insulin could save people with diabetes vindicated his optimism.

In 1922, the year that Frederick Banting and Charles Best published their astonishing paper about the isolation of insulin and first treated a human patient, the Rockefeller Foundation established the Committee for Research in Problems of Sex. The preeminent grantees supported by the committee would over the next twenty years discover many of the sex hormones and how they shimmy, shimmy, shake with one another in the endocrine dance. The improved understanding of ovulation and menstruation ushered in the birth control pill, fertility treatments, and a variety of miscarriage interventions.

The dance—and thus, in a sense, life itself—begins in the nose. Early in embryonic life, cells from the nose develop that later will secrete gonadotropin-releasing hormone, GnRH, a sexy beast that other hormones will follow onto the dance floor. As the embryo develops, these GnRH-secreting cells soon migrate to their final destination, a walnut-sized gland at that base of the brain that serves as the intersection between the nervous and endocrine systems, the junction of pain and pleasure. Not until 1980 did the monkey researcher Ernest Knobil at the University of Pittsburgh and his colleagues delineate the precise role of the hypothalamus and GnRH, which they described in two back-to-back *Science* papers.

Knobil and his team demonstrated how GnRH controls the onset of puberty and the monthly cycle of ovulation. In one experiment, the researchers destroyed the GnRH-producing region of the hypothalamus in seven adult female rhesus monkeys. Through implanted catheters, they pulsed in doses of GnRH for six minutes each hour for up to five months. As expected, the GnRH "urged on" (the meaning of hormone) a neighboring gland, the pea-sized pituitary, to send out follicle-stimulating hormone and luteinizing hormone, two biochemical cheerleaders that communicate directly with the gonads. With the ovaries urged on by these two hormones, collectively known as gonadotropins, the monkeys ovulated normally.

The menstrual cycle relies on a hormonal feedback loop that operates like a thermostat, turning the heater on or off as the temperature drops below or rises above a set point. The hypothalamus functions as the thermostat, with the pulsing of GnRH acting as the furnace. Hormones secreted by the pituitary gland and the ovaries drive the temperature up or down, completing the loop.

Great variation occurs in the length of a menstrual cycle, but on average, every twenty-three to thirty-five days, a woman will start a new period. Ovulation times also vary (to the dismay of many couples who have trusted the rhythm method of birth control), but it roughly occurs two weeks before the last period. For the sake of simplicity, doctors often have instructed patients that, on average, a cycle lasts twenty-eight days and ovulation occurs at day 14.

Eggs do not just pop out of ovaries. Each of the four hundred or five hundred eggs a woman will ovulate in her lifetime must survive a perilous yearlong voyage inside a follicle, the cluster of cells that protects it. Scientists turn to militaristic language to describe the arduous passage a follicle makes from "recruitment" to "selection" and, finally, "dominance."

After a follicle beats the fierce competition and wins dominant status, the hypothalamus pulses GnRH in such a way that the pituitary gland pulses follicle-stimulating hormone. The developing dominant follicle itself then pumps out increasing levels of estrogen, the superstar of the female sex hormones. Under the influence of estrogen, the uterine lining balloons to ten times its normal size. Estrogen also tells the hypothalamus to pulse GnRH, which prods the pituitary gland to spit out a large bolus of luteinizing hormone, the very "LH surge" detected by ovulation predictor kits on sale at supermarkets.

Drenched in luteinizing hormone, the dominant follicle releases its egg, which, if all goes well, will sweep into the fallopian tube in search of sperm.

The emptied follicle does not just disintegrate and disappear. Rather, it morphs into a corpus luteum, a cholesterol-filled yellow body that secretes yet another critical hormone, progesterone. Like estrogen, progesterone at first helps fluff up the uterine lining and even leads to the development of structures that help the embryo attach. As progesterone levels increase, the symphonic score crescendoes and the uterus prepares for the invasive trophoblast, turning the soil to bricks.

If no embryo implants, the lining sheds, causing menstruation and the hormonal dance begins anew. But if implantation proceeds, the placental trophoblasts secrete human chorionic gonadotropin, the hCG that home pregnancy tests detect. Just as luteinizing hormone nourishes the follicle, hCG nourishes the corpus luteum and "rescues" it from self-destruction.

The reproductive endocrinologist Bruce Lessey, an implantation authority based at the Greenville Hospital System's Center for Women's Medicine in South Carolina, told me that the Wilcox study about the optimal time of implantation holds the key to understanding luteal phase deficiency and miscarriage. As he put it, "Patients who don't implant on time don't get a timely rescue of the corpus luteum and then they lose the embryo because of ovarian neglect." At the unforgiving gambling table of reproduction, then, the very ovary that gives life can take it away.

A bizarre study published in 1972 dramatically elucidated the critical contribution made by the ovary's corpus luteum and its progesterone production. A team led by Arpad Csapo, a researcher at Washington University in St. Louis who laid the groundwork for development of the abortifacient RU-486, removed the corpus luteum from twelve pregnant women. As Csapo and coworkers explained, three of the women had ovarian cysts, while the other nine obstetrically normal women wanted to abort and have their tubes tied. Seven patients who had the surgery between day 42 and 57 after their last menstrual period all aborted, while the five patients who had the operation between day 52 and 74 of gestation did not. So until about the eighth week of gestation, the corpus luteum and the progesterone it supplies makes or breaks a pregnancy.

Georgeanna Jones, an ob-gyn who specialized in reproductive endocrinology at Johns Hopkins University, in 1949 first described luteal phase deficiency, and researchers have been arguing about it ever since. "I'm pretty convinced it happens, but we don't have a good way to diagnose it," Danny Schust told me. Schust, who studies implantation and runs the recurrent miscarriage clinic at Harvard Medical School's Brigham and Women's Hospital, echoed an opinion I heard from many in the field.

Jones, who with her husband later would pioneer in vitro fertilization in the United States, studied ninety-eight infertile women over 255 menstrual cycles. Because body temperature, controlled by the hypothalamus, spikes when a woman ovulates, Jones had each woman chart her temperature. Jones also took endometrial biopsies and checked progesterone levels via a biochemical marker found in the urine. She found dramatically different rates of luteal abnormalities with these different tests — from 13 percent who had inadequate luteal function based on temperature charts to 50 percent who had abnormal function based on the biopsies — but Jones persuasively documented the link to infertility.

The next year, Arthur Hertig and John Rock, working with R. W. Noyes, described an improved way to date the stage of a woman's menstrual cycle with an endometrial biopsy. To this day, most clinicians consider a modified version of their endometrial dating the best test for luteal phase deficiency. But because different labs read the biopsy results differently, tremendous confusion exists about whether a woman actually has a luteal phase deficiency. This lack of consensus, in turn, has made it difficult to make sense of clinical trials that evaluate progesterone and other hormonal interventions. Further complicating matters, a study published in 1994 by a team headed by Michael Soules, a prominent reproductive endocrinologist at the University of Washington in Seattle, found that measuring blood levels of progesterone at three different times and then pooling the results better diagnosed luteal phase deficiency than did the endometrial biopsy.

Many clinicians regard the use of progesterone to treat luteal phase deficiency as the single most controversial miscarriage treatment. "If you want to get a group of reproductive endocrinologists yelling at each other, just bring that up," said Soules. "It's a crazy area in our field." Soules told me that not only do disagreements exist about how best to diagnose the problem, but it can occur sporadically. Endometrial biopsy, he added, also causes physical pain in many women and is expensive to decipher. "It has served us well over the years, but it's relatively crude," he said. Soules said that he diagnoses luteal phase deficiency with pooled progesterone levels and then uses the endometrial biopsy only to evaluate whether a progesterone treatment has corrected the problem.

Controversy similarly surrounds the question of how many women have luteal phase deficiency. Soules, who once wrote that it "may be the most common ovulatory abnormality in women" and that it was "probably grossly underdiagnosed," said it occurs so frequently in women who do *not* have reproductive problems that it clouds the impact in women who do. In a 1996 study, Mary Stephenson, who treated Marian Anderson, helped clarify this point. Stephenson analyzed 197 couples who had at least three or more consecutive miscarriages without any evidence of a chromosomal abnormality explaining the loss. Based on endometrial biopsies, she found that 34 of these women, or 17 percent, had a luteal phase deficiency—the exact same number who had antiphospholipid syndrome. But whether progesterone helps remains a guess.

At least thirty clinical studies have evaluated whether progesterone can prevent miscarriages. In 2003, Richmal Marie Oates-Whitehead, an ob-gyn epidemiologist at the Royal College of Paediatrics in London, sorted out the often conflicting results of these studies with an exhaustive examination of the best of these trials. Pooling the results from fourteen studies into a meta-analysis that allowed them to evaluate far more patients than otherwise possible, Oates-Whitehead and coworkers found that in 1,098 women who received either progesterone or a placebo, the treatment produced no significant difference in birth rates. The only hint that progesterone might have helped came from three relatively ancient studies—one from 1953 and the other two from 1964—of women who had had three or more consecutive miscarriages.

It surprised me that the only studies of progesterone and recurrent miscarriage that Oates-Whitehead cited were so old. I asked her why she thought no researchers effectively addressed the question in four decades. "I think people stopped doing progesterone studies because they didn't get sexy outcomes," Oates-Whitehead said. "Nothing was happening."

Oates-Whitehead's perspectives deserve close attention—and not just because she carefully analyzed the entire body of scientific literature on the subject. When I spoke with her in 2003, Oates-Whitehead, thirty-four, had experienced ten miscarriages herself. To her own surprise, she still held out hope that she would become pregnant and carry to term. "I had a patient who came in who had thirteen miscarriages, and I thought, There's no way I'm going to do that," she said. "Here I am at ten. It's completely different when you're there. There is no logical reason why I keep trying." (She has never used progesterone, but not because she doubted its effectiveness; rather, she does not believe she has an implantation problem.)

In practice, many clinicians prescribe progesterone based on shaky diagnostic criteria and the conviction, bolstered by decades of use, that it will not cause serious side effects in either women or their babies. "I'd be first to admit it's kind of circular logic," Soules told me. "You think you see something, you diagnose, you treat, and you have a certain amount of success. You can convince yourself, but you can't really in the strongest sense of medical evidence prove it." Soules also pointed out what happens when he diagnoses a patient with luteal phase deficiency and then explains that no studies have proven the worth of taking progesterone supplements. "Often they say, 'Then I have nothing,'" Soules explained. "They think for a minute and say, 'Why don't we just do that?'"

The overlap of miscarriage and fertility problems adds another real-world aspect to this debate. "In today's fertility practice, if someone has luteal phase deficiency and it's not diagnosed, it will eventually get treated," Soules said. Women who have fertility problems typically will first receive Clomid, which both works against estrogen and leads to increased production of luteinizing hormone and follicle-stimulating hormone. As a result, the ovaries release multiple follicles in one cycle. Multiple follicles equals multiple corpora lutea and, logically, higher progesterone levels. Some clinicians use Clomid to treat luteal phase deficiency, but it has a serious drawback. Clomid also blocks estrogen's effects elsewhere, preventing the uterine lining from thickening—working at cross-purposes with progesterone—and derailing the process that makes cervical mucus hospitable to sperm.

When women need a bigger gun than Clomid to induce ovulation, they can inject follicle-stimulating hormone (which comes with or without luteinizing hormone). After injection, progesterone levels skyrocket. "You overwhelm the system," said Soules. He told me that he had never seen a case in which these injections thinned uterine lining, but pre-scribing them to treat luteal phase deficiency amounts to using a flame-thrower to start a campfire. Women treated with these gonadotropins also run the risk of ovulating several eggs, which can lead to twins, triplets, and higher multiples.

To clarify once and for all whether progesterone can help a woman with luteal phase deficiency carry a baby to term, researchers would have to stage a large, well-designed study at many clinics. But the pharma-ceutical industry has no financial incentive to fund such studies because the drug already has FDA approval. And, for researchers, the question has little intellectual cachet, as the underlying biology has received intense examination. As Soules told me, "I don't think there's much more to learn about the corpus luteum and progesterone production."

An end to the confusion likely will start to come when researchers can develop a better test to diagnose luteal phase deficiency. Recently, two groups have made progress on that front. Yale University's Harvey Kli-man has developed what he calls the Endometrial Function Test, and he has registered the name with the U.S. Patent and Trademark Office in the hope of selling it. The test measures two proteins that regulate the re-ceptiveness of the uterine lining. To assess the test's value for miscarriage patients, Kliman teamed with Vancouver's Mary Stephenson, who plans to send him four hundred endometrial biopsies: three hundred come from patients who visited her clinic while the other hundred come from women who have no miscarriage or fertility problems.

A new technique to study genes may provide another window into the uterine lining. Because hormones and the chemical signals that produce them travel from one place in the body to another, biologists describe their movement in terms of streams. In the case of progesterone, the hy-pothalamus is upstream and the uterine lining is downstream. To see all the way upstream to the source, scientists analyze genes. Humans have an estimated thirty to forty thousand genes, and they constantly flick on and off, working in concert to produce the proteins that drive biological processes, be it hormones and reproduction, the firing of a nerve cell to move a muscle, or the delivery of oxygen to lung cells. In the late 1990s, scientists discovered a way to place thousands of genes on a grid, each one labeled with a colored marker that displays which actors play a role in a specific process.

South Carolina's Bruce Lessey in 2002 published the first such massive analysis of the changes in gene activity that occur between the beginning and the middle of the luteal phase. Working with colleagues at the University of Delaware, Lessey put twelve thousand genes on a grid and, from that, began to ferret out the main actors responsible for creating a receptive uterus. One day in the not too distant future, Lessey hopes this research will lead to a highly specific test to diagnose luteal phase deficiency.

On September 11, 2001, shortly after the World Trade Center attack, Marian Anderson once again checked the luteinizing hormone levels in her urine, the test that turns positive at ovulation. "My stupid little stick came back at peak about a week earlier than I expected," she recalled. "I called my husband and said, 'The world's coming to an end! You've got to come home!'" The next month, she learned that she had become pregnant for the fifth time since the birth of her two-and-a-half-year-old son.

On Thanksgiving, Anderson began to spot. "Oh my God, I'm miscarrying again," she feared. The next Tuesday, she and her husband went to see Stephenson for an ultrasound. "I said, There's not going to be anything there." As the image came up on the screen, Stephenson found a heartbeat. "Everyone in the room seemed stunned," recalled Anderson.

Worried about the slight risk of miscarriage from amniocentesis, Anderson and her husband decided not to check their baby for chromosomal problems. But when she had reached her eighteenth week, they submitted to a detailed ultrasound scan to make sure everything was OK. They noticed that the technician repeatedly kept making a measurement. "What's wrong?" her husband asked.

The technician had found an abnormally large "nuchal fold"—a thickening around the nape of the neck that can indicate Down syndrome. After much deliberation, Anderson had an amnio, and, at twenty-two weeks into the pregnancy, she and her husband learned that their baby was chromosomally normal. On May 22, 2002—after suffering through four miscarriages, seeing eleven doctors, collecting two and a half feet of medical literature, and enduring a level of anguish that has no measure—Marian Anderson delivered her second healthy son.

I asked why she thought she carried to term this final time. The progesterone and heparin had helped, she believed, and she put much stock in her naturopathic regimen, too. But then she also looked at me in the eye and said, "I have no idea. Only God knows."

At the recommendation of her doctors, who worried about her antiphospholipid syndrome and other underlying health issues, Anderson requested a tubal ligation. When we met—her new baby was just fourteen months old—she told me she wanted another child. "If I was to win the lottery tomorrow I would hire a surrogate and have another," she said. "If I won a smaller amount, I'd adopt."

So much for not wanting children.

Other pregnancy-related hormones besides progesterone also have enticed miscarriage researchers as potential treatments. Several studies evaluating injections of human chorionic gonadotropin (including one completely fraudulent one, later retracted) assert that it might correct abnormalities in the follicular phase.

The most careful analysis of this question, published in 1994 by Roy Farquharson and Siobhan Quenby of Liverpool Women's Hospital in England, randomly assigned hCG or a placebo to eighty-one women who received care from the miscarriage clinic at Women's Hospital in Liverpool, England. Both the treated and control groups had an identical, astonishingly high success rate—86 percent—indicating that hCG offered no benefit. But an odd detail surfaced in the women who had a history of irregular periods and did not receive hCG: They carried to term only 40 percent of the time. Such "subset" analyses do not prove anything, but they do raise intriguing questions for further studies. Making the finding more curious still, it tied into another hormonal disorder linked to miscarriage.

Upon ultrasound examination, the most common abnormality that investigators find in women who recurrently miscarry is a "string of pearls" around the ovaries known as polycysts. Such polycystic ovaries have received intense study from fertility researchers, as they often exist in women who have aberrant levels of luteinizing hormone coupled with irregular periods or none at all. But researchers have struggled to tease out how this abnormality connects to miscarriage.

In 1990, Lesley Regan cowrote a study that reported a five times higher miscarriage rate in women who had elevated luteinizing hormone levels. This research set the stage for a study conducted at the St. Mary's Recurrent Miscarriage Clinic between 1992 and 1995 which investigated whether treatment could prevent miscarriages in women who had poly-cystic ovaries and high levels of luteinizing hormone. The controlled trial recruited 106 women who had had at least three consecutive first-trimester miscarriages but no evidence of antiphospholipid antibodies or other underlying problems.

The study's control group received either a placebo or progesterone suppositories. The menstrual cycles in the women in the treated group were aggressively manipulated with a barrage of hormones, including GnRH, follicle-stimulating hormone, luteinizing hormone, human chorionic gonadotropin, and progesterone. But after three years, re-searchers found that the heavy hormone stimulation offered nothing, nor did the progesterone suppositories alone.

Surprised by their negative results, the researchers reviewed the ul-trasound scans from more than two thousand women they saw between 1991 and 1999 and discovered that 40 percent had polycystic ovaries. The same research team earlier calculated that "normal" women had poly-cystic ovaries at only about half that frequency. But a further analysis re-vealed no connection to recurrent miscarriage. The researchers compared 233 pregnant women who had polycystic ovaries to 253 pregnant women who did not. Women in both groups had miscarried at least three times previously. In both groups, six out of ten women carried to term.

Yet these studies did not distinguish between women with polycystic ovaries who have clinical symptoms connected to the string of pearls — a condition called polycystic ovarian syndrome, or PCOS — and those who do not. With PCOS, the link to miscarriage becomes stronger. In addition to ovulation problems, a direct result of the hormonal imbalance, about one-third of PCOS women have excessive body and facial hair, an indicator that their bodies overproduce testosterone and other "male" hormones, which normally appear in females at low levels. Similarly, the male hormones can trigger outbreaks of acne. Many women with PCOS are obese. Many have difficulty properly using insulin, the hormone the body relies on to process sugars, and it rises to high levels. The prevalence of diabetes in this group also jumps to seven times that of healthy women.

The largest studies done to date of pregnant women with PCOS estimate miscarriage rates of between 40 percent and 60 percent, but with the wide range of symptoms that define this syndrome, questions still outnumber answers. Obesity itself, for example, appears to cause higher miscarriage rates. Still, trials of drugs that attempt to create a more normal hormonal environment in pregnant women who have PCOS have had promising results. In particular, two separate studies published in 2002 reported that metformin, which helps the body use insulin, significantly lowered miscarriage rates in women with PCOS. Neither, however, had a randomized, placebo-controlled, double-blind design.

Bruce Lessey, the South Carolina–based clinician who specializes in implantation, told me he has had some early success in PCOS patients using letrozole, an estrogen-blocking drug developed to treat breast cancer which also induces ovulation. Letrozole, he contends, may have a "revolutionizing" impact on both miscarriage and infertility patients, as it has two critical benefits over Clomid: letrozole does not thin the uterine lining—a potential cause of pregnancy loss—or change the cervical mucus. But, once again, no well-designed study yet has proven that letrozole can safely help women become pregnant and carry to term.

In May 2003, after reviewing the current scientific literature, the United Kingdom's influential Royal College of Obstetricians and Gynaecologists issued a treatment guideline to couples who had had three or more miscarriages. The Royal College advised women (except those who have diabetes or thyroid disorders) to steer clear of hormonal miscarriage treatments. Progesterone and hCG "should only be used in the context of randomized controlled trials," the report declared. The Royal College also reiterated the findings from St. Mary's on polycystic ovaries, advising that luteinizing hormone offered nothing. And they urged clinicians to resist the temptation to prescribe these unproven treatments.

Now add to these cautionary words the possibility that a hormonal intervention to prevent miscarriage could cause serious harm to mother, baby, or both. In fact, one hormonal miscarriage treatment did.

7

REALLY?

Trudy Merzbach miscarried when she was about thirty years old, an event that still reverberated in 2003, the year she celebrated her eighty-second birthday. Merzbach was four or five weeks along when she lost what would have been her first child. "I wanted it so badly," she said. "I was a complete mess and I fell apart." To recuperate, she left her husband in New York and went to visit her sister in Maryland, who then had a toddler. "It was good, and yet it was the worst thing," said Merzbach. "I was in the midst of a family."

As it turned out, Merzbach and her husband, Martin, in 1951 had a baby girl and then in 1952, a son. Her daughter, Fran, remembered with terrific clarity the car ride in the mid-1960s during which her mother revealed her miscarriage. With her father driving, Fran, then in her early teens, rode in the front seat and pretended that she had the wheel, a trick her parents devised to prevent their daughter, who was prone to motion sickness, from becoming nauseated. Trudy and her son rode in the back seat. As father and daughter wheeled the car past Farleigh Dickinson University in Teaneck, New Jersey, Trudy explained that she had lost a baby before Fran's birth. "I'd always been secure in my position as the oldest child, and when mom said she had a miscarriage before me, it was sort of like being hit by something," Fran told me. "The world wasn't the way I thought it was."

Nor was the world the way Trudy Merzbach then imagined it, the miscarriage just a painful memory that had no lasting consequence to her or her children. "It's funny that at the time it seemed the only significance was that it meant I wasn't actually the first," said Fran. "I didn't see it as a foreshadowing of a major factor in my life."

Shortly after Trudy Merzbach told her children about her miscarriage, doctors at Boston's Vincent Memorial Hospital saw the first cases of a rare cancer that altered the way the public and physicians would view hormones taken during pregnancy.

Between 1967 and 1969, doctors at Vincent Memorial, part of Harvard University's medical school, diagnosed six women between the ages of fifteen and twenty-two with a cancer of the vagina called clear-cell adenocarcinoma. One of the patients, a sixteen-year-old girl, died, and several of the others underwent surgeries to remove their vaginas and uteri. When the doctors reviewed the history of adenocarcinoma at their hospital they found that it had occurred only twice between 1930 and 1965, and never in a woman under twenty-five.

In 1969, a mother of one of the girls told Howard Ulfelder, the chief of gynecological services at the hospital, that she had a hunch what caused the cancer. "When I was pregnant with her, the doctor put me on stilbestrol because I had lost one pregnancy," she said. "Could that have anything to do with it?"

Stilbestrol, a trade name for the synthetic estrogen known as diethylstilbestrol, or DES, became a popular miscarriage treatment after Olive and George Smith, a prominent husband-and-wife team at Harvard University, reported in the late 1940s that the drug could prevent miscarriages and other pregnancy complications. An infamous advertisement that ran in a 1957 issue of the *American Journal of Obstetrics and Gynecology* captured how wondrously some viewed the drug. The ad for desPLEX, a version of DES made by the Grant Chemical Company—one of the drug's many manufacturers—featured a photo of a wide-eyed infant, index finger in mouth. "Really?" read the text. "Yes . . . desPLEX® to prevent ABORTION, MISCARRIAGE AND PREMATURE LABOR." The ad went on to recommend desPLEX "for routine prophylaxis in ALL pregnancies," noting that this formulation of DES contained "vitamin C and certain members of the vitamin B complex to aid detoxification in pregnancy."

Ulfelder dismissed the mother's suggestion that DES could have caused the tragic cancer in her daughter years after the fact. But Ulfelder and his junior colleague, the ob-gyn Arthur Herbst, soon linked several more cases of young girls with adenocarcinoma to their mothers having taken DES,

In April 1970, Ulfelder, Herbst, and the pathologist Robert Scully published a report in the journal *Cancer* that described these six cases as well as another one treated at a different Massachusetts hospital. But the little-noticed *Cancer* paper made no mention of potential causes, as the Harvard group wanted to make a rock solid investigation of their suspicions. Yet their informal surveying of patients left them with little doubt. When questioned, a second mother told Ulfelder she had taken the drug, and he also found two more cases of the rare vaginal cancer in young women (one in California and the other in Mexico), whose mothers had taken DES. Herbst, first author of the *Cancer* paper, separately had a startling conversation with the mother of the one girl who had died from the disease. When Herbst told her they suspected DES might have caused the adenocarcinoma, she said, "You can stop your study. I took DES."

Herbst, Ulfelder, and David Poskanzer conducted a carefully designed study that compared the mothers of their patients to mothers who had not taken the drug. The results made the case that DES had caused clear-cell adenocarcinoma in seven young women they had studied. "It was a terrible thing and a terrible tragedy for the young women who got it," Herbst, who later moved to the University of Chicago, told me. "When a kid sixteen, seventeen is essentially castrated, it is horrible."

Shortly before the *New England Journal of Medicine* published the study, Herbst took a copy of their paper to Olive and George Smith. "I knew them very well and thought they were wonderful," said Herbst, who himself had prescribed DES for high-risk pregnancies. "They were very upset, and gave me all their records to contact people they had given DES to."

The report in the April 22, 1971, *New England Journal*—which included a commentary from the epidemiologist Alexander Langmuir, who said the study was "of great scientific importance" and raised "serious social implications"—received little media attention at first. Save for the *Wall*

Street Journal running a one-paragraph story in its daily roundup of "What's News" and the Associated Press putting out a short notice that ran in several papers, many major dailies, including the *New York Times*, ignored the report, as did the network news programs. By that August, however, with DES-linked cases of adenocarcinoma mounting, the story had ballooned to the point that *Time* magazine ran a two-page accounting titled "Hormonal Time Bomb?"

Martin Merzbach noticed the *Time* story and recognized the name diethylstilbestrol. Wasn't that the drug he used to pick up at the pharmacy when Trudy was pregnant with Fran?

After Trudy had her miscarriage, her doctor advised her to come to him as soon as she became pregnant again. "I'll give you something to prevent miscarriages," he said. In the winter of 1950, Trudy followed his advice and took injections at his office of diethylstilbestrol for the first three months after testing positive for pregnancy. She then switched to DES pills, the ones Martin would fetch at the pharmacy. In January 1951, when Trudy gave birth to Fran, she was "absolutely convinced" that DES had allowed her to carry to term.

When Trudy became pregnant again in 1952, she specifically requested DES, but her doctor said that she probably did not need it. "I was deeply disappointed," Trudy said.

Reading the old scientific studies about DES, dating back to the first promising report in 1946, is like reviewing the transcripts of cockpit recordings recovered from the black box after an airplane crash. It should become required reading for anyone who promotes a miscarriage intervention.

George Smith, a gynecologist at the Boston Lying-in Hospital, and his wife, the Harvard University biochemist Olive Smith, pioneered the use of DES in pregnant women. The Smiths reported in 1946 that they had tested DES in one thirty-six-year-old pregnant woman with diabetes who had preeclampsia during her two previous pregnancies, one of which ended in a stillbirth. The Smiths showed that, just as they had hoped, DES boosted the production of progesterone, which they theorized would prevent late-pregnancy "accidents." The woman gave birth to a healthy eight-pound baby boy, and suffered no preeclampsia. They noted that "there has been no evidence of harmful effects." The Smiths further suggested that DES might have many other powers. "The progesterone stimulating properties of diethylstilbestrol make it an equally logical agent for the prevention of accidents in early pregnancy," they concluded.

In 1948, Olive Smith presented findings gathered from 117 obstetricians in 48 cities across the United States who had followed what she called the "Smith and Smith schedule" of treating pregnant women with DES. They divided treated women into different groups, depending on whether they had "threatened abortions" (bleeding or cramps between weeks 6 and 21), infertility problems, two or more miscarriages, or complications of late pregnancy. In all, their study had 632 case reports. Each group of women—except those who previously had miscarried four or more times or had had three or more previous premature deliveries— gave birth to healthy babies between 70 and 87 percent of the time.

This evaluation did not compare the results to a control group. Olive Smith, however, did attempt to bolster the contention that DES worked by citing results from other studies that evaluated women who recurrently miscarried. In particular, she highlighted the famous study published by Percy Malpas in 1938 on "abortion sequences." Based on "the known incidence of abortion in the British Empire and of the accidental and recurrent factors involved," Smith noted that Malpas had calculated that a woman who had miscarried three times and became pregnant again had a 27 percent chance of carrying to term. Another study of women in the same situation had a "spontaneous cure rate" that was even lower—about 16 percent. Olive Smith asserted that the high success rates among the women who took DES "cannot possibly be ascribed to chance," and for women who repeatedly miscarry, "seem to establish beyond any reasonable doubt the value of stilbestrol therapy."

With the benefit of hindsight and the cool dispassion that the passing of decades provides, these arguments seem labored, even naïve. The original study described one woman and thus meant next to nothing. The analysis of 632 cases divided into different groups involved an impressively large number of DES-treated pregnancies, but it was a far cry from a randomized, placebo-controlled study. The supposed linchpin, the comparison to other studies of recurrent miscarriages, further clouded the truth: as several subsequent studies have shown, women who miscarry three times and become pregnant again carry to term, with no intervention, up to 70 percent of the time. And confusing all of the DES results presented by the Smiths was that they studied women who began their treatment at different times; because most miscarriages occur early, the women who started DES further into their viable pregnancies had a higher likelihood of carrying to term. Safety concerns largely focused on such trivial side effects as nausea and headaches, as well as the possibility that some clinicians had not followed the Smith and Smith schedule and thus had given patients too high a dose of the drug. Olive Smith ended her 1948 discussion of safety with an aside that, in the harsh light of retrospect, seems glib: "A few patients, in whom therapy had been discontinued after their danger periods had passed, voluntarily began taking stilbestrol again because they claimed that they felt so much better when taking it," she reported enthusiastically.

At a 1949 meeting of the American Gynecological Society, the Smiths reported findings from a controlled study they had done that specifically looked at whether DES could prevent the complications of late pregnancy in women who had become pregnant for the first time. The ambitious study, conducted at the Boston Lying-in Hospital, compared 387 treated women to 555 untreated controls. Most women began treatment between the twelfth and sixteenth week of pregnancy, by which time most miscarriages would already have occurred. Women who took DES, they found, had less preeclampsia and gave birth to heavier, longer babies, an indirect measure of their health.

After the presentation, the Smiths' colleagues held a discussion with them. No one questioned the safety of DES in either mother or child, and only one, William Dieckmann from the University of Chicago, had the temerity to note that the Smith study did not use a placebo in the controls, which could have biased the results.

Dieckmann four years later, at the same meeting, presented results from his own carefully controlled study of DES that compared a whopping 840 treated women to 806 controls. DES had no effect on the incidence of miscarriage, preeclampsia, or even the baby's birth size. The Smiths went to great lengths to explain why his results did not match their own. "Our experience with the use of stilbestrol continues to be satisfactory and to confirm our previously reported clinical results," said George Smith at the 1953 meeting. "We have never claimed it was a panacea, but after ten years of careful study and observation of patients with bad and even hopeless prognoses at the onset of pregnancy when stilbestrol was started, we are convinced that it has reduced the complications of late pregnancy and saved many babies." Olive Smith asserted that colleagues "frequently misrepresented" the Smiths' findings. "To anyone who has carefully read our papers it will be apparent that this report by Dr. Dieckmann and his associates is no exception in this respect," she said. "We have never said that it should be given to all women during pregnancy. . . . We feel sure that the difficulties that have arisen in this controversy would be greatly reduced if a clearer understanding of the rationale were more prevalent." The response of others in the audience included more testimonials of DES's worth, including one Floridian physician who said, "As a former Bostonian, I would be entirely lacking in civic loyalty if I had not used stilbestrol in my private practice."

Important differences in trial design did make it difficult to compare the Dieckmann study's results to the ones obtained by the Smiths. As often happens in science, the noise from this technical debate drowned out Dieckmann's negative findings, and clinicians continued to prescribe DES to pregnant women, although the drug's popularity steadily waned. By the time that researchers linked DES to adenocarcinoma, Trudy Merzbach was one of between 2 million and 10 million pregnant women—no precise figure exists—who had taken the drug. And other, much more common harmful effects of DES soon would surface in female babies, like Fran, who had received the synthetic estrogen while still in the womb.

The Food and Drug Administration in November 1971 issued a drug bulletin that advised clinicians to stop prescribing DES to pregnant women. Ten months later, Arthur Herbst and his coworkers again stunned the medical community and the public: they implicated DES as the cause of vaginal and cervical abnormalities, including odd ridges and malformed glands. And if DES interfered with the proper development of the vagina and cervix in the embryo, then, logically, it might have had a negative effect on the developing uterus and fallopian tubes, too. Raymond Kaufman, an ob-gyn at Baylor College of Medicine in Houston, began examining this possibility in 1974 as part of a nationwide study of DES's effects spearheaded by the U.S. National Cancer Institute. "It was a matter of deductive reasoning," Kaufman explained to me.

Embryos begin life with the potential to become either female or male. If no male chromosome exists, the embryo will destroy the male apparatus and develop the female one, which starts as a pair of tubes called müllerian ducts, which abut the kidney. Between six weeks and sixteen weeks after conception, the müllerian ducts zip together, but only partially, leaving two separate fallopian tubes that branch off like the arms of a Y. The fused portion forms the uterus, the cervix, and the upper two-thirds of the vagina. Given that DES appeared to cause changes during the formation of the vagina and the cervix, the uterus thus became the next logical place to look.

Kaufman and his colleagues examined the uteri of sixty young women whose mothers had taken DES while pregnant. To view each womb, they first inserted a tube through the vagina, and then injected a dye into the uterus and fallopian tubes. This procedure, a hysterosalpingogram, allowed an X-ray to capture an image that revealed whether the uterus had the appropriate shape and the tubes could freely pass fluid. "When we started to do the hysterosalpingograms, sure enough we started to see bizarre findings," said Kaufman. "Originally, we were very surprised."

In 1976, Kaufman presented their findings at an ob-gyn meeting. Of the sixty young women they studied who had been exposed to DES in utero—a group that would become known as "DES daughters"—a staggering forty had unusual upper genital tracts as compared to women who had hysterosalpingograms as part of infertility evaluations. Medical records revealed that the five women whose mothers took DES late in pregnancy (after eighteen weeks gestation) had fewer and less severe abnormalities. But most startlingly, twenty-one of the women had narrow uteri that took the shape of a T rather than branching into the proper Y. "It will be extremely interesting to observe, in the next several years, the pregnancy outcome in patients with abnormal uteri," concluded Kaufman.

Kaufman's audience immediately recognized the implications of this study. In a formal discussion after his presentation, one colleague presciently said, "I believe this is one of those unusual papers which guarantees historical and medical importance, will be quoted often, and will stimulate many new discoveries to questions we have not even imagined yet."

In April 1977, a month before Kaufman and his colleagues published their landmark study, Pat Cody met in Manhattan with a group of women who took DES, and they decided to form DES Action, a grassroots organization to spread the word about the drug and its potentially harmful effects.

Cody first became pregnant in 1954. "I was thirty-one, which was very late in those days," she said. A few months into the pregnancy, she miscarried. A neighbor who had had her own pregnancy problems suggested that Cody see a doctor who supposedly had "a great new medicine." Cody took the advice, and when she became pregnant in May 1955, she swallowed her DES pills for seven months, steadily increasing the dosage every few weeks as per the Smith and Smith schedule. In February 1956, she gave birth to a healthy baby girl, and a few months later Cody and her husband opened Cody Books, which became a well-known bookstore on Telegraph Avenue in Berkeley, California.

I asked Cody whether she thought at the time that DES had helped her carry to term. "Oh my gosh, yes," said Cody. "Of course. Absolutely. That's a problem we have now. Many mothers naturally feel terrible about this and tell their daughters you wouldn't be here without DES."

Cody in 1979 helped found the "DES Action" newsletter. That same year, her own DES-exposed daughter had an ectopic pregnancy and her fallopian tube ruptured. She subsequently developed severe endometriosis, which Pat attributed to DES. Her daughter had a complete hysterectomy at age thirty-four.

Trudy Merzbach subscribed to "DES Action" and bought a separate subscription for daughter, Fran, who had little interest in the subject. Fran, who had become a radio journalist, moved frequently from city to city, and the newsletter followed her from place to place. Eventually, she started to read it, and she became convinced that she might have problems conceiving and carrying to term.

Fran married at thirty-eight and quickly sought help from a reproductive endocrinologist. "I raised the alarm very early," said Fran, whose married name is Howell. "At thirty-eight, I didn't have a lot of wiggle room." A hysterosalpingogram revealed that Fran had a T-shaped uterus.

Fran started with Clomid to help her ovulate, and then moved up to injections of Pergonal, artificial insemination, and, finally, a whole slew of hormones required for in vitro fertilization. She didn't see the irony in eagerly taking hormonal treatments to become pregnant after her mother's hormonal treatment had harmed her. "It wasn't that I had blinders on," said Fran. "I just didn't connect the dots."

Her mother, however, did, but held her tongue. "I didn't want her exposed to that," said Trudy. "But how can you tell a child who wants a child not to do it? I caused the problem."

In June 1991, doctors transferred two embryos into Fran. She and her husband decided that whatever happened, they had reached the end of infertility road. Neither embryo implanted.

It turns out that DES causes clear-cell adenocarcinoma of the vagina in about one out of every thousand women exposed to the drug in utero. This devastating disease propelled the dangers of DES into the spotlight, and, given the public's fear of cancer, added an extra dimension to what Roy Pitkin, the former editor of *Obstetrics & Gynecology*, called the "long and convoluted saga." But the tragedy of the rare adenocarcinoma has overshadowed the frequency with which the drug caused T-shaped uteri in Fran and other DES daughters.

Soon after tying DES to adenocarcinoma, Arthur Herbst and his coworkers set up a registry to track every known case of the cancer in DES daughters. As of May 2002, the Registry for Research on Hormonal Transplacental Carcinogenesis had 750 cases, only two-thirds of which had a clear link to DES. Herbst told me that in his career, he has seen no more than three dozen patients with this cancer.

Raymond Kaufman's group continued to study uterine abnormalities, and in a 1983 report on 676 DES daughters—more than ten times as many as they initially assessed—problems occurred about 40 percent of the time, but T-shaped uteri still occurred in 30 percent of the women. Kaufman subsequently participated in several massive reviews of the reproductive fate of DES-exposed women. In October 2000, Kaufman and his colleagues published what they predicted would close the book on this question, as the average age of a DES daughter had reached forty-five, marking the end of the reproductive years. This remarkable study gathered information from 443 women whose mothers took part in Dieckmann's famous 1950s study of DES, roughly half of whom received a placebo, providing an excellent control group to compare the drug's impact. The researchers also queried more than 3,300 DES daughters and 1,000 controls, many of whom took part in the nationwide study sponsored by the National Cancer Institute in the mid-1970s.

DES daughters more frequently miscarried, especially during the second trimester, and nearly twice as many reported not becoming pregnant after trying for a year. Exposed women who had identified uterine problems were seven times more likely to have experienced infertility.

A few small studies have reported successful surgical repair of T-shaped uteri, but Kaufman, for one, remained unimpressed. "I think that's a waste of time," he told me. "It's an operation that doesn't do anything." His conviction rested on a stunning finding, included in his 2000 report, culled from reviewing reproduction in 1,269 DES daughters. Although they had more fertility problems and miscarriages than the controls, nearly 75 percent of the DES daughters eventually became pregnant, and of those who did, 85 percent carried to term at least once. Although this study did not specifically separate out women with T-shaped uteri, Kaufman's smaller, earlier studies did, and found that slightly more than half, at an average age of thirty years old, had had a live-term birth versus about three-fourths of the DES-exposed women who had no detectable abnormalities, again indicating that the abnormality caused reproductive problems, but did not prevent most women from having a baby.

Concern about the harm caused by DES has extended well beyond the T-shaped uteri, adenocarcinomas, and other problems suffered by DES daughters. Studies have shown a slightly increased risk of breast cancer in mothers who took the drug. Some studies have investigated whether DES harmed males exposed in utero, and though one abnormality occurs more frequently—noncancerous cysts on the testicles—no serious problems have surfaced that mirror the compelling evidence of harm that researchers have found in DES daughters. Many researchers also have explored whether the drug affected grandchildren of women who took DES, but no convincing third-generation effects have yet to surface.

Adding a final insult to DES's legacy, a 2003 meta-analysis combined the results of five studies, including Dieckmann's, done between 1950 and 1955 and involving a total of nearly 2,500 women. DES, the analysis concluded, clearly *increased* the risk of miscarriage.

In the midst of their increasingly aggressive and expensive fertility treatments, Fran Howell and her husband explored adoption. Because they had different religious backgrounds and were both nearing forty, adoption agencies gave them the cold shoulder. So before doing in vitro fertilization, the Howells decided in 1991 to place newspaper ads seeking a pregnant woman who wanted to find a good home for her baby. "It was empowering," said Fran. "Things were so out of our hands. Medically you just do what they say, you have no control."

They set up a separate phone line, and, said Fran, "every time that phone rang it was just frightening." But they quickly hit it off with a woman who called, a restaurant worker who already had a child and worried that another baby would force her onto the welfare rolls. By the time Fran went in for the ill-fated embryo transfer, they already had decided to adopt. "When in vitro didn't work, I didn't feel as bad," said Fran. But her tortuous journey to become a mother had more heart-stopping curves ahead.

Fran went with the woman to each of her prenatal visits, and they became close. "It was a really good experience for us, and I think the world of her," said Fran. When the woman gave birth to a healthy baby girl, both

Fran and her husband were at the hospital. "The minute they put her in my arms I knew she was ours," said Fran. "She's such a good fit."

They took their new daughter home in November 1991, but they soon received the call that adoptive parents dread. "I've made a mistake," the birth mother said. "I want my child back." Apparently, the woman's own mother had pressured her to renege on the agreement. The birth mother took them to court and a January hearing date was set. "It was the most emotionally difficult thing I've ever been through," said Fran.

Certain they would lose in court, Fran had difficulty going into the baby's room and cuddling her. "You go in there and hold that baby because she needs to be held," Fran's husband told her. "Her needs come first." Fran's voice choked up when she told me this story, as though it had happened weeks ago, not thirteen years earlier. Fran of course did rock the baby, surrounded by presents for her that they left unopened through the Hanukkah and Christmas holidays, uncertain that, come January, she would still be their daughter.

The Howells prevailed in court, and Fran stays in touch with her daughter's birth mother, sending her photos of the girl three times a year. "We are so lucky to be her parents," said Fran.

Diethylstilbestrol was first seen as a wonder of medicine for its supposed ability to help women bring babies into the world, only to stain medicine's reputation when it became clear that it caused those very babies grievous harm. Some have pointed fingers at the Smiths and their acolytes, violating the physician's maxim, "First, do no harm." But singling out the Smiths as culprits distorts the truth.

The Smiths had their faults. They glibly dismissed criticisms. Even considering the standards of the time, they made claims that required leaps of logic. The true believers who followed the Smith and Smith regimen deserve blame, too. But players besides the Smiths and their supporters made tragic mistakes. Without question, the Food and Drug Administration failed. In the wake of the adenocarcinoma discovery, it has raised the hurdles that drugs must clear before winning approval for use in pregnant women. The tangled relationship among the pharmaceutical industry, doctors, and the public also contributed to the uncritical approval and overprescription of DES, as two Columbia University researchers noted in their 1952 report of DES's failure to prevent "threatened" abortion:

> The public has been so frequently told of the virtue of this drug through articles appearing in lay journals that it now requires a courageous physician to refuse this medication. The mass of pharmaceutical literature, extolling the wonders of this drug, has also rendered most practitioners amenable to his patient's demands. This situation, together with the understandable desire to do something positive toward rescuing a teetering pregnancy, has resulted in the widespread use of DES in threatened abortion.

But there remains another, more difficult factor both to see and to accept, and understanding it could help prevent similar catastrophes from recurring. Deciding to do nothing, in an informed way, often constitutes the most prudent way to do something. Women and men who want babies, especially those who have tried and failed, would benefit if they recognized how their intense desires can lead them to take unnecessary risks. It bears repeating again and again and again. Most women who miscarry, even three or four times, will carry to term if they become pregnant again. More than half of women who have T-shaped uteri will become pregnant and carry to term. So most any intervention, from standing on one leg and reciting the Gettysburg Address to taking an unproven hormonal treatment, will, most of the time, appear to work. And as happened with Trudy Merzbach, Pat Cody, and the millions of other women who took DES during pregnancy, they may logically end up in the delivery room praising an intervention that, years later, they will come to curse.

This danger does not mean that people should avoid all miscarriage interventions. But the DES debacle warns that, as much as possible, people struggling to have a baby would do well to evaluate first whether they have an underlying biological problem and then, if offered a treatment option that supposedly has a proven record as safe and effective, to ask, from every imaginable angle, Really?

8

ANATOMICALLY INCORRECT

LESLEY REGAN, THE OB-GYN WHO HEADS THE RECURRENT Miscarriage Clinic at St. Mary's Hospital in London, in the early 1990s performed a hysterectomy on a seventy-five-year-old woman who had complained of "something uncomfortable coming down below." The woman's pelvic muscles had weakened, causing prolapse, a condition in which the uterus drops into the vaginal canal. During the surgery, Regan realized that the woman had two uteri that joined at one cervix.

When Regan told the woman of her discovery and explained that this abnormality was linked to miscarriages, fertility problems, and premature labor, the woman gently replied that she had never miscarried, and had had six sons who each weighed eight pounds or more at birth. "She probably had a healthy suspicion of me, who she perceived as being a relatively young doctor with lots of theories about how things should be," Regan said.

Regan tells this story to make the point that uterine abnormalities do not necessarily cause problems. Abundant evidence backs this conclusion. But, once again, a close look at the picture reveals more gray than black and white. As studies of DES daughters with T-shaped uteri indicate, an abnormality of the womb can lead to a wide spectrum of reproductive fates: it often increases the difficulty of becoming pregnant and carrying to term, but then many of these women do give birth to healthy babies—and no clear line separates them from those who do not.

Estimates in the 1980s of the incidence of uterine abnormalities led to a ridiculous range of conclusions—from 1 in 10 women to 1 in 1,600—a good indication that no one had a clue. But the discrepancies have narrowed as clinicians have improved their diagnostic techniques and refined their definitions of the various problems. An excellent overview published in 2001 by a Greek and Belgian team combined results from several well-done studies and revealed that uterine malformation occurred in 4.3 percent of nearly 3,000 normal, fertile women. A separate analysis of more than 4,500 women who had recurrent miscarriages, in contrast, revealed that 12.6 percent—nearly three times as many—had abnormal uteri, which suggests a strong link.

In addition to the T-shaped uterus, a half dozen other uterine "anomalies" that have odd-sounding names—didelphys, bicornuate, septate, and arcuate—exist, and they all occur during the developmental process that transforms the conceptus into either a male or a female. Reproductive organs develop from the müllerian ducts, the two tubes that begin in the embryo as separate entities, and then, if no Y chromosome exists, partially fuse together to form the upper portion of the vagina, the cervix, the uterus, and the fallopian tubes. At one extreme, a female may have only a single müllerian duct, creating one "horn," which physicians appropriately call a "unicornuate uterus." If the two ducts do not fuse properly, two completely separate "didelphic" uteri can form—sometimes with two cervixes and even two vaginas—or the top of the organ can jut down, forming a heart-shaped, two-horned "bicornuate" uterus. If during fusion the embryo does not properly absorb the walls of the müllerian ducts as they become one, it can leave a septum, like the "septate" cartilage that divides the nostrils; in a variation on this defect, a slight septum creates an arc at the top of the uterine cavity, or an "arcuate" uterus. The Greek-Belgian team again lumped together several studies, this time analyzing 1,392 women who had uterine abnormalities, and found that septate uteri occurred the most frequently, accounting for a little more than one-third of the anomalies, with bicornuate a close second (26 percent), and arcuate third (18 percent). On average, only about half of the women in these studies gave birth, with the arcuate group ranking the highest (66 percent).

Different surgeries attempt to correct these anatomical problems. Surgery done through the vagina can fix a septate or arcuate uterus, while bicornuate and didelphic uteri typically require cutting through the abdomen, as with a C-section. Some studies report astonishing success rates, including one of bicornuate uteri, which said that 289 women, who lost 70 percent of their pregnancies before the surgery, had a live birth rate of 85 percent after correcting the problem. Other studies have shown that surgery has no impact. As often occurs in the surgical field, no study has used a randomized control group of matched, untreated women with the same abnormality. Patients, many of whom join drug studies and willingly allow chance to decide whether they receive the treatment or a placebo, basically have a greater reluctance to roll the dice when it comes to going under the knife. Surgical intervention by and large thus is based on woolly data and beliefs, rather than on hard scientific evidence.

During the past decade, a movement called "evidence-based" medicine has gained much momentum. Led by physicians in the United Kingdom, the movement fesses up to medicine's shortcomings: all too often, procedures and treatments become popular because of personal experience, tradition, and the beliefs of individual clinicians when the doctors should be relying on serious studies that have validated a procedure's worth. Evidence-based medicine, which has spawned its own eponymous journal and centers at leading universities, aims to help clinicians cull the mountains of scientific literature for the most compelling data. The movement also proselytizes the value of randomized, controlled trials.

But when it comes to surgery for uterine anomalies, convincing evidence will remain in short supply. The ob-gyn May Backos, a strong proponent of evidence-based medicine and a key member of Regan's team at St. Mary's Hospital Recurrent Miscarriage Clinic, launched a controlled, randomized study of surgery for septate uteri in 2002. "It's been slow to recruit," Backos told me when I visited her in July 2003. I asked her what "slow" meant. "It's more than a year now," she said. "I haven't got anyone yet."

At twenty-nine, two years into her marriage, Mary Skarsgard became pregnant by accident. "I get pregnant very easily," Skarsgard told me nine years later. "That's one of the blessings and the curses." At five weeks, she miscarried. "I didn't give it much thought," she said. Later that year she became pregnant for the second time, which again ended in a five-week miscarriage. She had her third miscarriage the next year, 1995, yet another embryo that stopped growing at five weeks.

At the suggestion of her physician brother-in-law, Skarsgard saw Mary Stephenson at the recently opened Vancouver recurrent miscarriage clinic. A biopsy of Skarsgard's uterine lining revealed a luteal phase deficiency, so Stephenson prescribed progesterone suppositories to bring her ovulatory cycle into sync. A hysterosalpingogram showed that Skarsgard had a septate uterus, but Stephenson did not think removing it would help. "I was a nonbeliever," Stephenson told me. "Does it intuitively make sense? Most likely, you're not going to have three or more consecutive losses because of a septate uterus. They're just not going to implant."

In 1996, Skarsgard became pregnant again, and the baby's heart beat on an early ultrasound. But the embryo stopped growing at six weeks, and Skarsgard miscarried again. "I went through a major depression," she said. "It was silly that I didn't get help." Adding to her blues, each time she became pregnant, as an extra precaution she suspended her workout routine at their home gym. "I love being active," said Skarsgard, an athletically built, yet petite, elementary school teacher. Becoming pregnant and repeatedly miscarrying, she said, "was taking parts of me and who I was."

In the summer of 1996, Skarsgard and her husband, Paul, needed a break from the ordeal, and vacationed in Europe, where they enjoyed not trying to become pregnant. When she returned, she still had irregular bleeding, so they sought help from a second fertility specialist recommended by her brother-in-law. The specialist suggested that he could safely remove most of her septate uterus, which might help solve her problem. This surprised Skarsgard, as it contradicted what Stephenson had said, but she had the operation.

Skarsgard restarted progesterone treatments, and soon became pregnant for the fifth time, but again, the embryo died at six weeks. An analysis of the embryo showed that it was a boy with a normal number of chromosomes.

Still determined to have a child, Skarsgard added aspirin to her treatment when she became pregnant in 1998, but she had exactly the same fate: a chromosomally normal boy that died at six weeks. Later that year, she returned to Mary Stephenson, who for the first time diagnosed moderate levels of antiphospholipid antibodies in Skarsgard's blood. She began injecting heparin, in addition to taking aspirin and progesterone, but miscarried again that year and the next, bring her total losses to eight.

Before performing a dilation and curettage to remove the six-week-old embryo of her eighth miscarriage, Stephenson viewed Skarsgard's uterus with a hysteroscope, and to her astonishment, the embryo had implanted on a nubbin of the septum that the surgery had not removed.

The embryo's location made Stephenson rethink the process of implantation. Why would it implant on the septum and not the fluffy endometrium? she asked herself. The more she thought about it, the more she became convinced that a septum could lead to miscarriages. "You think the endometrium is a wonderful, lush lining that's very inviting to fertilized eggs," she said. "Actually, it's a very hostile environment and prevents implantation except in this window. It's the opposite of what you think. My original theory is a bunch of crap. The window of opportunity over the septum is more inviting than the lush lining. So there may be a preferential susceptibility to implantation on the septum."

Stephenson noted that her hypothesis is unproven, but she removed the septal remnant. Over the course of her eight miscarriages, Skarsgard had evaluations that included an endometrial biopsy, a hysterosalpingogram, a hysteroscopy, measurement of antiphospholipid antibodies, and karyotyping of three fetuses (each of which had normal chromosomes). She had taken heparin, aspirin, and progesterone. Stephenson hoped that removing the nubbin, finally, might allow Skarsgard to cross the natal finish line. And to nudge the odds in Skarsgard's favor a little more, Stephenson also suggested that she try one other experimental treatment, intravenous immunoglobulin.

In September 2000, Skarsgard became pregnant for the ninth time. "Everything was great," she said. When she had some early bleeding, she decided to take a leave from her job and go on bed rest, another unproven intervention. Week after week, everything checked out fine. Amniocentesis detected a boy with a normal complement of chromosomes.

Mary and Paul bought a crib, and an interior designer friend helped set up the room. "We kept on getting the go-ahead," she remembered.

As she approached May 2, her date for a scheduled cesarean section,

Skarsgard noticed that the baby wasn't moving as much. "He was big, and I was small," she figured. As a precaution, Mary and Paul on March 28 went to the doctor for a stress test on the baby. "Perfectly fine," she said. "We were really happy everything was going so well." That night, she did not feel the baby move. She tried to shrug it off. *I went for a stress test and everything was fine*, she told herself. *He probably was sleeping.* In her dreams that night, the baby was moving.

When she awoke, she sensed that something was wrong. Skarsgard had an ultrasound scheduled for that day, and she told Paul he had better come along. Her mother joined them. When the technician jellied her belly and started to sway the ultrasound wand to and fro, Skarsgard immediately asked her to check for a heartbeat.

"OK, we'll get to that," the technician said.

"No, check the heartbeat," Skarsgard insisted.

A few moments later, the technician dashed out of the room.

"He's died," Skarsgard announced.

"No, no, she just went to get some more gel," Paul said.

"I know he's dead," said Skarsgard. "Stop kidding yourself."

Skarsgard, a devout Greek Orthodox Catholic, does not remember much from the next few minutes, other than saying to her mother, "I know there's a reason for this, there's a reason why God took him."

The doctors shuttled the family to a grieving room. "I was losing my mind," Skarsgard said. A doctor then informed them that they could not perform a C-section for two days. "We begged and pleaded with them to do it earlier so he could find his peace," remembered Skarsgard. But the doctors would not budge. "In the long run, I appreciated it because for two days, we were together," she said.

On Friday, March 30, 2001, Skarsgard gave birth to Christopher Lloyd, who had died in utero from a perforated bowel. "Paul was standing beside me, and I said, 'You go first and tell me what it's like,'" remembered Skarsgard. "Paul was hanging over the bed sobbing. I had never seen him like that. He kept on saying, 'We have a little boy. We have a little boy.'"

Skarsgard held her son, who weighed exactly four pounds. "He was just perfect," she said. They dressed Christopher in an outfit they had brought along, and they took photographs holding him.

Mary and Paul stayed in the hospital ward with Christopher for the next two days. "I'm so happy we got Christopher," she said. "In the end, I was thrilled at the hospital. My mother-in-law looked at me like I was on drugs—which I was—but I was *so* happy. I was a mother to him."

The Skarsgards had a funeral for their son. Skarsgard's mother objected. "You don't have a funeral for a baby who died who hadn't lived," her mother said. Her parents had also tried to convince her not to see the baby. But Skarsgard felt she had to do both.

Mary also came to a profound understanding of why she had clashed with her mother about Christopher's fate. "My mom had lost a baby at about five months after my birth," she said. "She never saw the baby and never knew whether it was a boy or a girl. It was just incinerated. For her, this was bringing up all these things. But she held him, and I think it brought closure for her."

The process brought closure for Mary and Paul, too, who decided at the hospital to adopt. "We can't go through this again," Paul said.

Mary Skarsgard emotionally bottomed out the night before they buried Christopher and a few of his things in a white coffin. "I kept thinking, He's going to be so lonely," she said. "I wanted to go with him. I wanted to die myself."

Skarsgard keeps a picture of Christopher beside her bed. "He's part of us," she said. "I pray for him every night." She carries a picture with him in her wallet, too, which she held up for me to see. He looked lifeless, but I noticed his head of hair, the blanket that wrapped him, and how essentially human it seemed to take comfort from the picture, as unusual as it was. I asked her why she thought God took him. "Because he was a perfect angel," she said.

During her two days in the hospital after giving birth, Skarsgard said she could hear the other mothers on the ward with their crying newborns. "None of it bothered me," she said. "I had had my baby."

Skarsgard came to terms with her fate in a way that deeply moved Stephenson. "It changed me," Stephenson told me.

From Skarsgard's perspective, after eight miscarriages, she had had a child.

. . .

When I entered an unused examination room at the St. Mary's Hospital pregnancy clinic in London to meet Sasha Jelic, I immediately laughed. Jelic had a crooked smile that said, Yeah, I know, I look silly. Sitting on the tip of the seat of a standard office chair, she leaned far back, her legs extended straight. The posture reminded me of a sunbather, lying on a chaise longue and sipping a drink with a cocktail umbrella in it. A sunbather with a gibbous belly. "I'm twenty-eight weeks now," she said, holding up crossed fingers on both hands.

Jelic, thirty-six, explained to me that since the thirteenth week of her pregnancy, she had placed herself on bed rest because of her "incompetent" cervix, which means the uterine door to the vaginal canal opens too early, frequently causing second-trimester miscarriages. Jelic, who grew up in Yugoslavia, had two miscarriages in 2001, at around the nineteenth week of her pregnancies. Both times, she had received the one treatment for a weak cervix: cerclage, a surgery commonly performed through the vagina—either as a purse-string suture or with surgical tape—which, theoretically, should bar the door until the baby has come to term (at which point the suture is removed).

More than four decades after clinicians started routinely tying up incompetent cervixes, cerclage continued to polarize the ob-gyn community. In March 2002, James Harger, an ob-gyn at the University of Pittsburgh, published a critique of cerclage in which he called it a "crude, archaic procedure." That same year, *Obstetrics & Gynecology* ran a more formal "evidence-based analysis" by Harger that reviewed the abundant literature on cerclage, which led him to go so far as to suggest that the procedure "may be unethical."

I contacted Harger, who recently had retired after specializing in recurrent miscarriage for thirty years. He told me he found the scientific literature about cerclage "a mess." Although he had performed many cerclages during his career, he said he became "immensely critical" after carefully evaluating the evidence supporting the procedure. "I'm a little bit like the reformed smoker," he said.

As foggy as the benefits of cerclage may be, no dispute exists about its dangers, which include the possibility of cervical infection, cervical tearing that can occur if a woman goes into labor without having had the sutures removed, and the general risk that accompanies any anesthesia. Harger stressed one other less obvious risk: it leads clinicians to ignore other, potentially more relevant explanations for recurrent miscarriage.

Other than infection, factors that cause the cervix to weaken largely remain a mystery—some studies have shown links to other uterine anomalies, exposure to DES, and even antiphospholipid antibodies. But a clearer understanding of the condition has emerged to upend the textbook definition of cervical incompetence. Cervical incompetence wrongly implies that a cervix either functions or does not. A multicenter study sponsored by the U.S. National Institutes of Health of nearly three thousand pregnant women, which Harger contributed to, used transvaginal ultrasound to measure their cervixes at about twenty-four weeks of gestation. The researchers, who published their findings in a 1996 issue of the *New England Journal of Medicine,* revealed that the shorter the cervix, the greater the likelihood of a preterm delivery. So cervical problems occurred on a continuum, leading Harger and others to begin referring to "cervical insufficiency" rather than "incompetence."

Because no clear-cut definition of cervical insufficiency exists, no firm diagnostic criteria exist, although for a time, many hoped that an ultrasound measurement of a shortened cervix would provide the answer. "It sounded so good, and it didn't pan out," said Harger. The absence of a valid way to detect the condition makes it impossible to determine its frequency or whether an intervention works.

Traditionally, clinicians have used a patient's history as the main diagnostic: women who previously have had an unexplained second-trimester loss are classified as being at high risk for cervical incompetence. Harger noted that studies of women who have a history of preterm delivery reported that between 10 and 35 percent had a subsequent one. Flipping that fact on its head, 65 to 90 percent of women who doctors classify as cerclage candidates do not actually benefit from the surgery.

Adding clouds to the tempest, different studies evaluate different types of cerclage. In an elective cerclage, a woman chooses the surgery because of her past losses. An urgent cerclage attempts to take advantage of the supposed insight provided by a transvaginal ultrasound measurement of the cervical length. Between the twentieth and twenty-eighth week of pregnancy, a normal cervix measured with ultrasound typically stretches to 3.5 centimeters in length. (A fingertip roughly spans one centimeter.) In 10 percent of women, the cervix shortens to 2.5 centimeters or less in this time frame, and several studies have evaluated the worth of cerclage in such urgent situations. Finally, clinicians sometimes perform an emergency cerclage if, in the absence of labor, the opening of the cervix dilates more than 1.5 centimeters or so.

Scrutiny of cerclage's value first intensified after two separate research groups published results of their randomized controlled trials. One study of 194 women found that elective cerclage did not alter the preterm delivery rate, while the other, which involved 504 women, had similar results—but also discovered that those who received the stitch had *more* first- and second-trimester miscarriages. The researchers recruited different women for their studies: one excluded volunteers who had had a second-term miscarriage of a live fetus, while the other limited its participants to women who had had second- or third-term miscarriage. Critics concluded that neither study actually targeted the women most likely to benefit from cerclage.

A large international study of elective cerclage led by the U.K.'s Medical Research Council in collaboration with the Royal College of Obstetricians and Gynaecologists recruited 1,292 women whose obstetricians were uncertain about whether they should have cerclage. This study, published in 1993, again showed no benefit of elective cerclage, except in the 107 women who had had at least three second-trimester miscarriages. In this subgroup, the preterm delivery rate plunged from 32 to 15 percent in those who received the cerclage. Critics of this study ripped into it for not properly selecting participants.

Researchers have tested urgent cerclage, which relies on the diagnosis of a shortened cervix, in two much smaller, but well-designed, studies. At the annual meeting for Maternal-Fetal Medicine in 2000, Orion Rust and colleagues from Lehigh Valley Hospital in Pennsylvania reported that they had randomly assigned sixty-one women who had shortened cervixes to receive cerclage or no treatment. The researchers did not find any statistically significant differences in either group, with about one-third giving birth before thirty-four weeks and four babies dying in one group and three in the other.

At the same meeting the next year, a Dutch group led by Sietske Althuisius reported findings from their study that compared cerclage and bed rest to bed rest alone in thirty-five women who had shortened cervixes before twenty-seven weeks of gestation. The nineteen women who received the cerclage all carried to term and their babies survived. Of the sixteen women who received only bed rest, seven gave birth preterm and three of the babies died. Althuisius and his coworkers argued that, once again, different entry criteria in the two studies led to the different outcomes, but with so few participants, it becomes difficult to separate the effect of cerclage from the forces of chance.

The Pennsylvania team also presented an update at the conference. By then, the researchers had evaluated fifty-five women in the cerclage group versus fifty-eight who did not receive treatment. Their earlier findings held: cerclage did nothing. In a 2001 publication of their results, Rust and his colleagues offered a trenchant analysis of the difference between their study and the Dutch one, concluding that they simply had more patients—and thus more believable evidence. They did allow that, in the future, researchers might develop diagnostic criteria that reveal a subset of women who do actually benefit from cerclage.

Harger sung the praises of this study to the hilt. "They did this not at a Harvard or a Yale, but a dinky little hospital in Pennsylvania." It excited him so because it gave the lie to the frequently heard complaint from clinicians that they cannot recruit patients to a controlled cerclage study. He ran into such a roadblock when he tried to organize a study in the 1990s with the help of the nationwide network of doctors who ran the trial that evaluated transvaginal ultrasound and cervical length. "They all said we will never persuade any of the doctors to do this, and, secondly, the lawyers will kill us because this had become the established standard of care," recalled Harger. (In medicolegal terminology, a "standard of care" refers to what a prudent physician would do in a specific situation.)

Finally, emergency cerclage, used in the dire situation in which a cervix begins to dilate early, has no randomized, controlled studies to support its use.

A meta-analysis of 2,175 women published in September 2003 found no benefit to either elective or urgent cerclage. Save for the unusual situation in which a woman, like Sasha Jelic, has had two unexplained second-trimester losses, the authors of this study cautioned that "the skeptic would not offer cerclage at all."

As for Sasha Jelic, despite cerclage having failed twice before—including one that caused such a severe infection that she ended up in the intensive care unit shortly after she lost the baby—she chose to have a cerclage with this pregnancy, too. Diagnosed with antiphospholipid syndrome, she also took baby aspirin and daily heparin injections. Since week 13, she had put herself on a program of bed rest, which her father, a retired physician, had recommended. "He's had lots of discussions with doctors back home, and they say it relieves the pressure on your cervix and it will help," said Jelic. She paused for a moment, and said, "Dr. Regan's research has shown bed rest doesn't help." Jelic shrugged.

Jelic had no way of knowing which factors led her to make it to twenty-eight weeks, a point at which she had an excellent chance of giving birth to a healthy baby. "It's really hard for me to tell what it is that's helping," she said. "I've been greatly encouraged that I should walk." Another shrug. "But I keep sitting funny. I lie in taxis like this going to the clinic and coming home. Now it appears my cervix has begun to open. I keep praying."

I asked her whether she was religious. "No," she said. "But I keep saying, 'God, please.'"

Her sister, it turns out, also had an incompetent cervix and spent seven months in the hospital on bed rest. "If you want something, I say no price is too high," said Jelic. "It's really a short period of time. Now I say, 'A couple of weeks, a couple of weeks.'" She said she and her partner of eighteen years declined to find out the sex of the baby. "They say it helps you get through labor not to know," she said.

On September 30, 2003, Sasha, at full term, gave birth to a six-pound, two-ounce son. A few days later, I received an e-mail from her son, Sam, which included pictures and this short note: "I have arrived safe and sound."

I like the incongruity of Sasha Jelic praying. The what-have-I-got-to-lose mindset drives many of the decisions that women who have miscarried make when faced with an unproven intervention. And this determination must assume some responsibility for propping up dubious practices.

From cerclage to uterine surgery, from hormones to immune treatments, the unknowns outnumber the knowns. The best clinicians understand this dilemma, and also recognize the vulnerability of patients who have miscarried. I do not second-guess doctors who submit to an informed patient's desire to try a surgical stitch, a septum removal, progesterone, or intravenous immunoglobulin. Sure, given the ambiguities of these treatments, they should be assessed in a clinical trial. Yet even Harger acknowledged the logic in recommending a cerclage in a patient such as Jelic. "I would really not be as strident about that," he told me when we discussed the specific situation. "The trouble is we get to the point where we say, 'It's just a cerclage, it's a purse-string suture with silk, I can do it in five minutes. It's a very simple operation.'"

It is easy to criticize doctors who have great enthusiasm for novel surgical procedures or experimental drug treatments. But individual physicians discover worthy interventions by such derring-do, interventions that ultimately prove safe and effective in well-designed studies. Harger and other evidence-based advocates of course understand this process of discovery, but, rightly I think, counter that off-label use of drugs and unproven surgical interventions, especially in patients desperate to have a baby, require a much more restrained approach than now typically occurs. They also push to understand the mechanism behind a supposed biological phenomenon: what, for example, physiologically happens to create a shortened cervix? "What we know is superficial," said Harger. "It's not grounded in molecular biology or genetics."

Harger said that strong cultural forces lead ob-gyns to embrace questionable interventions too often. "There's a whole tradition in ob-gyn where you compare women as their own controls," he said. "They'd say a woman had zero fetal survival, and with my cerclage she had a live birth." He did not spare himself this indictment, telling me the story of a pregnant woman who came to him with a yeast infection, whose cervix had dilated one centimeter, no cause for alarm. He cerclaged her. "That's my albatross," he said. "Guess what? She delivered at term. My partners said, 'Good call, Jim.' No one ever said that's not such a great idea." Patients who previously have miscarried also often arrive firmly convinced that they need a cerclage, he said, and resent the clinician who disagrees.

Then add in the emotionally charged atmosphere, with a distraught couple who finally secure a few precious minutes with the expert they hope can help solve their problem. "The secondary gain you get from ignoring scientific principles is seductive," said Harger. "The problem in all of miscarriage care is the emotional physician."

When I first met with Lesley Regan, she gave me some gimlet-eyed advice. "Be skeptical about people who are so vehement about their beliefs," Regan cautioned. "This is a field that attracts true believers." As with Harger, she well recognized the role that the patient played in this equation. "It's quite difficult to deal with patients who always want you to do something," she said. Adding it all together, it becomes that much more imperative for clinicians to acknowledge—forcefully, repeatedly, candidly—how much they do not know. As Regan summed up the field, "We are largely in the dark."

The fact that Christopher Lloyd expired in the womb did not influence the decision of whether Mary Skarsgard would give birth to him vaginally or via a cesarean section. Nature had made the choice for her. Skarsgard had a uterine fibroid, a benign tumor that postmortem studies have shown occurs in at least 20 percent of women, but shows up much less frequently on ultrasounds. Fibroids can cause pelvic pain and prolonged bleeding, and in the United States account for one-third of the hysterectomies performed in women who have yet to go through menopause. Under the influence of the surge of hormones released during pregnancies, fibroids can swell, preventing a vaginal delivery, which led Skarsgard to have a C-section.

Some evidence links fibroids to miscarriages, and some ob-gyns remove them in patients who have repeated pregnancy losses. Mary Stephenson told me she removes them only in the relatively rare instance in which they distort the uterine cavity, in which case they can interfere with implantation, which did not apply to Mary Skarsgard. And like many of her colleagues, Stephenson had deep misgivings about the few reports that claimed to reduce miscarriage rates by removing these fibroids.

The unconvincing miscarriage data reflect a deeper problem. Despite the frequency with which women develop fibroids, the quality of the research that evaluates various treatments has led ob-gyns to groan louder than they do about any other single topic I have examined. In 2002, researchers working with the Evidence-Based Practice Center at Duke University reviewed more than six hundred articles on fibroids. Only 10 of the 128 studies that involved surgical treatment had randomized patients. Their blistering critique concluded that "there is almost no high-quality evidence on which to base treatment strategies." That assessment becomes even more damning when you consider that, in the United States, surgeries to treat fibroids have become the second most common surgical intervention in women (C-sections come in first). "The thing that's striking to me is that fibroids are so common and such a big health issue, yet there's little research into what works and doesn't work," said Evan Myers, the ob-gyn and epidemiologist who headed the study.

A few studies specifically evaluated the impact of removing fibroids in women who previously miscarried, and all relied on a retrospective analysis. Such studies typically look back at hospital records and then compare treated to untreated patients. Where a *prospective* study diligently strives to reduce biases by choosing similar patients and then giving them either a treatment or a placebo, a retrospective study must make many assumptions about the two groups it analyzes. A retrospective analysis thus runs a substantially higher risk of apple/orange comparisons, as some critical distinction between the treated and control groups might not show up when reviewing patient charts. Piling several retrospective analyses together can mislead a field, as did several studies in the early 1980s that linked endometriosis (the growth of endometrial tissue outside of the uterus) to miscarriage. Controlled, randomized prospective trials later convincingly showed that no such connection exists.

An article in a 1997 newsletter from the Society for Obstetric Anesthesia and Perinatology explicitly discussed the shortcomings of retrospective analyses with specific, telling examples of how they can reach erroneous conclusions. A retrospective study asked whether women who received an epidural, the spinal injection of an anesthesia frequently given during labor, had more C-sections. The records did not indicate the amount of pain a woman felt before receiving the epidural. Logically, those in more pain would more frequently request this anesthesia, and the source of that pain, rather than the medication, might better explain why they needed C-sections.

As Mary Stephenson told me, "Retrospective studies aren't good enough."

After the Skarsgards' travails, women who knew their story, some nearly strangers, began to offer to carry a baby for them. Potential surrogates included a physician who worked with Paul's brother. The wife of Paul's brother offered too. Neither seemed right. Paul's brother later bumped into a woman at a wedding who inquired how Mary's pregnancy had gone and then asked whether she might help. Mary somewhat reluctantly agreed, but simultaneously pursued adoption on the side.

When Mary and Paul had in vitro embryos made, only one of three looked good, but doctors transferred all of them to the surrogate. One took. But then the woman phoned and said she had started to spot. "I thought, Yes!" remembered Mary. "I was so happy. This was great." Miscarriage means different things at different times.

Mary had never felt completely comfortable with the surrogate idea, and when the woman miscarried, they put their adoption plan on the front burner. Eight months later, they adopted a boy through a private agency. The birth mother, twenty-one, could not afford to have her child. "It was her wise decision," said Mary, who since has gone out to dinner with her. "She has come into our lives for a God-given reason. I will accept her and love her for the rest of my days. I think we were meant to have an adopted baby."

A few months after I met with Skarsgard in July 2003, she wrote me that she had had a tubal ligation, and said that she and her husband had no plans at the moment for more children. "We are very happy as a family of three," she wrote. By any measure, Mary Skarsgard, as much as anyone I had ever met, had come to terms with miscarriage.

PART THREE

HOPE

9

THE SKY ISN'T FALLING

IN THE SPRING OF 1893, THE DEVELOPER WILLIAM T. LOVE announced his grandiose scheme to build Model City, a utopian vision that would turn the farmlands just northeast of Niagara Falls, New York, into an industrial dreamscape. Love envisioned hundreds of manufacturers flocking to his Model City of up to 600,000 residents. The New York legislature had just passed a law that granted his Modeltown Development Corporation astonishingly broad powers to condemn property, and—crucial to his master plan—redirect water from the upper Niagara River, which fed the famous falls. The Love Canal, as it became known, would allow ships to move between Lake Erie and Lake Ontario, and would return water to the lower Niagara River via a new three-hundred-foot drop, creating a steady source of cheap, electrical power for nearby homes and businesses. "All telephone service, water, steam heat, electric power, street-railroad service, and gas are to be furnished to residents at cost," read a *New York Times* report of the announcement.

In a search for investors both stateside and abroad, Love aggressively and imaginatively advertised his Model City, even hiring brass brands to perform "Yankee Doodle," which he had revised with his own lyrics, which included these stanzas:

> Everybody's come to town.
> Those left we all do pity.
> For we'll have a jolly time
> At Love's new Model City.

Our boys are bright and well-to-do,
Our girls are smart and pretty.
They cannot help it, nor could you
If you lived in Model City.

When construction of the canal began in July 1894, two thousand people from across the state arrived on special trains to join in a celebration, which included oration from William T. Love, who predicted that completion of the project would take one year.

More than eight decades later, Anne Hillis composed her own verse about Love's Model City, a place where she had lived for thirteen years and had come to see as a "contaminated hell":

It, my soul, is ripped. It's being torn
apart! It hears the crying out,
It feels the anguish. The souls of so
many babies. "Redemption" is their shout,
I cry my tears. I beg my release
tiny souls made to stop.

In mother's womb, the chemicals came,
Our own inadequacy we did blame,
Now we know, the Corporate Murderers,
When their souls do pass,
The tiny ones, I pray with silence,
It will say "hush my own tiny one"
"God" is having his day.

By May 1979, when Hillis read this poem as part of her testimony to a New York State Senate committee, the canal that Love's "Yankee Doodle" ditty predicted "'twill make all very rich" had become infamous for making people sick. Most notoriously, pregnant women who lived near the star-crossed Love Canal supposedly had an increased rate of miscarriage, which gave pregnancy loss perhaps the most high-profile media—and political—attention it ever had received.

Love Canal became an internationally known symbol of the damag-

ing effects that disregard for the environment can have on future gener-
ations. It also played a central role in leading President Jimmy Carter to
propose the legislation that eventually became the U.S. Environmental
Protection Agency's Superfund, a federal program to clean up hazardous
waste sites. And it raised the public consciousness, just as the book *A Civil
Action* and the movie *Erin Brockovich* later would, about the difficulties that
communities face when they attempt to take corporations to task for en-
dangering their health.

Love Canal most likely did cause health problems, and the misbe-
havior of the various government bureaucracies deserved the outraged response of the residents, and then some. And those who broadcast this
disaster and keep its memory alive deserve society's thanks. But the history of Love Canal carries another discomfiting message, and it has to do
with miscarriage research.

Clusters of miscarriages, like clusters of cancers, have a unique power
to cause fear. But establishing cause and effect, to show in a scientific way
that a miscarriage occurred due to something in this environment, has
proved one of the most elusive endeavors in the field. Researchers repeatedly have failed to prove that what women eat, drink, inhale, absorb, or
physically experience presents a significant risk of causing a miscarriage.

Common sense dictates that a pregnant woman should avoid toxic
chemicals, cigarettes, bungee jumping, tall glasses of whiskey, many
medications, and certainly cocaine. Things that do not cause miscarriages
can harm a baby. But my own excavation of Love Canal's miscarriage controversy led me to the opposite conclusion from the one fixed in cultural
memory. The story of Love Canal, if it has any impact on how people think
about the risks of miscarrying, should *calm* fears. In the final analysis, the
link between miscarriage and the more than two hundred chemicals eventually discovered at the site proved as illusory as William T. Love's canal.

The many woes suffered by the Hillis family and their neighbors could be
traced back to William T. Love's bad luck. As tirelessly as this charismatic
entrepreneur tried to raise money for Model City, his timing proved dis-
astrous: an economic depression walloped the country in the mid-1890s,
and technological improvements made it relatively cheap to transport

electricity long distances from its source. By 1910, the Modeltown Development Corporation had foreclosed on its property. The would-be seven-mile canal ran a mere three thousand feet long and in places had been dug only ten feet deep. Parts of the rectangular trench became a summer swimming hole and a winter ice skating rink.

In the 1930s, the Hooker Electrochemical Corporation purchased the canal, which it used as a dumpsite between 1942 and 1952, burying, by its own estimates, 21,800 tons of chemicals in a decade. In 1953, the company sold the sixteen acres of land that included the dumpsite to the Niagara Falls Board of Education for $1, writing into the deed that it was not responsible for future harm caused by the buried chemicals. In turn, the Board of Education built an elementary school on the land and sold other portions to the city and a private developer. The former dump soon had about one hundred homes built along its banks.

Following unusually heavy rains and snowfall in the 1970s, residents who lived near the canal began to notice odd odors in their basements, and some discovered chemical sludge leaching through their walls. Children sometimes had burns and blisters on their hands after playing near the site, including on the school playground. Plants and pets mysteriously died. Some said they even had witnessed birds falling from the sky. In 1976, the *Niagara Gazette* began to report these oddities, which drew interest from a U.S. congressman, the New York State Department of Health, and the Environmental Protection Agency. After a private firm detected polychlorinated biphenyls in the soil—better known by the acronym PCBs—and a benzene compound, both cancer-causing agents, an EPA representative visited the site in September 1977. The EPA official observed rusted chemical barrels sticking out of the ground and could easily smell the chemical stench. His official report noted that three days later, his sweater still smelled. "Unhealthy and hazardous conditions exist," he concluded, noting the FOR SALE signs around many homes. By 1978, a grassroots activist organization had formed, the Love Canal Homeowners Association. In April 1978, the New York state health commissioner declared that Love Canal presented "an extremely serious threat to the health and welfare of residents" and ordered the first health studies. Come June, armed with scientific evidence showing that the site had at least thirty-eight chemical contaminants, the health commissioner issued an emergency declaration that ordered the Niagara County Board of Health to "abate the public health nuisance" by cleaning Love Canal and limiting access to the site.

This shocking tale remained under the national media's radar until August 2, 1978, when the health commissioner, in another emergency declaration, announced that Love Canal "presented a great and imminent peril" to residents living near the former dump. The trigger for this bombshell: A study by the health department of ninety-seven families showed a "significant excess" of miscarriage and birth defects in families who lived close to the site. According to the preliminary analysis, pregnant women in this neighborhood had a miscarriage rate of nearly 30 percent.

President Carter approved emergency aid for the area, and the state purchase of the homes of the 239 families "most immediately adjacent" to the site. The fevered pitch rose higher still in September, when the New York State Department of Health released the report "Love Canal: Public Health Time Bomb." The thirty-six-page report, its incendiary title printed in red type atop an apocalyptic aerial shot of the site, included a photograph of protesting residents with children holding placards that read PLEASE DON'T LET ME DIE and WE WANT OUT NOW! Three pages considered the miscarriage data, the same number that the report gave to analyses of chemical contaminants. By October, residents had filed more than eight hundred lawsuits against Hooker and various government agencies, demanding more than $11 billion in restitution. In December, the din grew louder still when the Department of Health discovered that the site also held dioxin, a known carcinogen.

Members of the Love Canal Homeowners Association who were not bought out by the state sought help from Beverly Paigen, a cancer researcher at Roswell Park Memorial Institute in Buffalo, who assessed the site's health hazards. Paigen found increased miscarriage rates well beyond the homes on the canal's banks. The Department of Health soon arrived at similar results, leading officials to call for a larger evacuation, but without outright purchase of the homes. The U.S. House and Senate soon followed with hearings in March 1979, which included testimony from Paigen and several outraged residents, Anne Hillis among them.

Hillis, who had lost one baby at the halfway mark and subsequently had a hysterectomy, detailed the many health ailments her ten-year-old son had suffered: asthma, abscesses in his nose, and depression. "I hate my life at Love Canal," she said. Citing Paigen's findings, she noted that one in four pregnancies had ended in miscarriage, "a rate far above the national average." She pleaded with the senators to understand the hopelessness, disillusionment, and fear that she and her neighbors felt. "Are we not Americans?" she asked. "I am a sick woman, nursing a sick child. My thoughts are, Will he live to have children? If so, will they be sick or deformed?"

Explosive stuff.

But from the outset the epidemiologic analyses that linked Love Canal to miscarriages made a thin case and, as the studies expanded to include more residents, the hypothesis became less tenable still, eventually disappearing altogether. The first study—the one that played a central role in propelling the Love Canal story from the front page of the *Niagara Gazette* to page one of the *New York Times*—rested on interviews conducted by the New York State Department of Health in a house-to-house survey. By August 20, 1978, a few weeks after the health department revealed the 30 percent miscarriage rate, it had sent interviewers armed with a detailed questionnaire to two hundred families who lived in a four-block radius of the landfill. The results from this survey, printed that September in "Love Canal: Public Health Time Bomb," showed that 22 percent of the pregnancies had ended in miscarriage. Already, the canal's ability to end pregnancy had weakened.

The researchers, cognizant that older women miscarried more frequently, broke the miscarriages down by age groups. For a control, they turned to the most authoritative study on the risk of miscarriage at various ages. Published by Dorothy Warburton and F. Clarke Fraser of Canada's McGill University in 1964, the study examined the outcomes in nearly seven thousand pregnancies and took the first close look at the relationship between maternal age and miscarriage. Using these findings as a benchmark, the New York State Department of Health scientists calculated the number of miscarriages they would have expected for five age brackets of pregnant women and then compared that to what their house-to-house surveys had found.

A cursory look at the evidence indicated that something frightening had taken place at Love Canal, where women experienced 1.5 times as many miscarriages as expected. Women who lived at the southern end of the dumpsite had lost 35 percent of their pregnancies, as compared to about a 15 percent miscarriage rate in the Warburton-Fraser study. But scientific results become increasingly less meaningful the more researchers make claims not based on their original theses and create sub-studies within the study. Scientists call it data dredging.

The seemingly high rate of miscarriage at the canal's southern end involved nine miscarriages out of thirty-nine pregnancies, a sample so small as to be statistically insignificant. Women up to twenty-nine years of age saw fewer than the expected number of miscarriages. But in the age bracket of thirty to thirty-four, six of nineteen pregnant women miscarried, more than twice the expected number. This loss became even more pronounced in the thirty-five-to-thirty-nine age bracket, in which eight of fifteen pregnancies did not go to term, again more than twice what they expected.

I asked Dorothy Warburton what she thought of the supposition that Love Canal caused miscarriages. After completing her graduate work at McGill, Warburton moved to Columbia University in New York City and earned the respect of her colleagues as one of the world's foremost authorities on the causes and incidence of miscarriage. "My reaction at the time was this was scaremongering, and these were not valid scientific studies," said Warburton, whose tussled, curly hair gives her a delightful, somewhat eccentric flair. She took exception to the notion that her studies could provide a control group for the Love Canal analysis. "You just can't extrapolate," she said. "No epidemiologist would say you could do that. It's using historical controls from a different era, different racial groups, and a different location, where they defined miscarriage differently. It's bad."

On the heels of the New York State Department of Health's miscarriage study and its October 1978 announcement that the increased pregnancy losses occurred only in women who lived directly adjacent to the canal, the Homeowners Association fought back with Beverly Paigen's analysis, which made even grander assertions based on skimpier data. As Paigen later would explain in congressional testimony, after she determined where clusters of miscarriages and birth defects had occurred and discussed her findings with older residents, they suggested that the problems overlapped with the location of the streambeds that used to flow from Love Canal before the homes existed. Paigen compared the number of miscarriages women had before they lived in these Love Canal "wet areas" with the number they had after moving there: they zoomed from 8 percent to 25 percent—results that, statistically speaking, had more than a 99.99 percent probability of *not* having occurred due to chance. She noted, too, that a number of women had experienced multiple miscarriages after having moved near a wet area, including one who had three miscarriages and a surviving baby born with three ears.

Paigen cautioned that her survey "suffered from several problems," including its reliance on memory rather than medical records. Still, she recommended that all women of childbearing age who wanted to have more children should be evacuated and then wait six months before attempting to become pregnant "to allow chemicals to be excreted from the body."

The New York State Department of Health followed up with a much more carefully done study, which compared families nearest to the canal with those who lived in areas that might have suffered from the chemicals traveling through streambeds and the like. This time, the researchers attempted to confirm memories of miscarriages with medical records. The findings hardly made a compelling case. Women who lived in homes on Ninety-ninth Street that abutted the canal had 1.5 times more miscarriages than expected from the Warburton and Fraser study and 6 times more than those in the neighborhoods a few blocks farther away. But on Ninety-seventh Street, which also abutted the canal, women had slightly *fewer* miscarriages than Warburton and Fraser predicted and about the same amount as their most distant neighbors.

Overall, of the 351 pregnancies that the researchers evaluated, 61 ended in an early loss, a miscarriage rate of 17 percent. If Love Canal led to miscarriage, the researchers concluded that only a "slight to moderate excess" occurred in a few specific regions. The researchers included the appropriate caveats, urging that their results "must be interpreted with great caution." The findings spurred the New York state health commissioner in February 1979 to urge residents living within twenty square blocks around the canal to relocate temporarily if a pregnant woman or children under two lived in the house.

The firefight between the government and the remaining families came to a head in May 1980 after the EPA reported that a scientific study done by an outside contractor revealed that eleven of thirty-six people tested supposedly had chromosomal abnormalities, a known cause of cancer, birth defects, and miscarriages. Paigen, reported the *New York Times*, "said the findings completed a cycle of proof" that the Hooker chemicals caused these maladies. Paigen reiterated her view that evacuation should occur immediately. Finally, on May 21, 1980, President Carter declared another federal emergency, with buyouts that paved the way for 710 families to leave the area for good.

Dorothy Warburton visited Love Canal with a team of scientists around this time to help calm the fears about the chromosomal data. "It was the most dreadful study," groaned Warburton, who said great concern existed that the residents would hold her group hostage, as had happened with two EPA officials. "We were just trying to convince them that this study wasn't true. When we talked to them and tried to reassure them, they didn't want to be reassured. If the refrigerator broke down, it was Love Canal. If the husband turned to drink, it was Love Canal."

That June, New York Governor Hugh Carey established a scientific panel to evaluate the various Love Canal studies. Led by Lewis Thomas, the Memorial Sloan-Kettering physician who became famous for his books (including *The Lives of a Cell*), the committee excoriated most every study and official body involved with assessing the potential harm caused by the Love Canal chemicals. The committee members agreed with the many criticisms that by then had surfaced of the chromosome study, "but feels even more strongly that such a poorly designed investigation as this one should not have been launched in the first place." In a backhanded compliment, they commended Beverly Paigen "as a private citizen" for attempting to evaluate the complex situation, but the report that she presented to Congress was "literally impossible to interpret" as it fell "far short of the mark as an exercise in epidemiology," they wrote. "It cannot be taken seriously as a piece of sound epidemiologic research, but it does have the impact of polemic." The New York State Department of Health's miscarriage data, they cautioned, "cannot be taken as more than suggestive." They concluded that the "scientific evidence, incomplete though it is, reveals no state of population damage justifying the terms 'imminent peril' and 'profound and devastating effects.'"

When the panel submitted its review in October 1980, Thomas wrote Governor Carey an unvarnished cover letter. "The Panel's recommendations attempt to assure that the circumstances which have resulted in inadequate science will not be repeated," wrote Thomas. "It may be too late to remedy the mistakes of the Love Canal experience; but there remains an opportunity to avoid a repetition of such mistakes in the future."

In 2003, I contacted Beverly Paigen, then a mouse researcher at the well-regarded Jackson Laboratory in Bar Harbor, Maine. More than two decades after the Love Canal contamination surfaced, Paigen still smarted from the Thomas panel's critique and what she viewed as other harassments inflicted upon her by the state of New York. "They were attacking me mercilessly," said Paigen, who charged that because of her Love Canal work, New York State had pulled the plug on her research grants and audited her income tax for the first time in twenty years. As conspiratorial as these complaints sounded, she struck me as thoughtful, rational, and more curious than defensive about the scientific questions surrounding miscarriage. She sent me a stack of scientific papers about her many studies that assessed the health impacts of Love Canal, not one of which looked at miscarriage. "The miscarriage data is some of the messiest data," she acknowledged.

Paigen had little doubt that the dumpsite presented health hazards to the community before she conducted any studies. "You only had to go there and smell the air and you knew there was something bad," she said. And just as she conducted her initial informal interviews with residents, a boy had kidney failure and died soon after playing in chemical sludge in a creek near the site.

Paigen studied several potential health impacts of living near Love Canal, mainly focusing on problems in children which she could measure: birth weight, growth rates, skin rashes, seizures, and learning disabilities. She even examined the health of the voles that lived in the area. She published scientific papers on all of these topics. "I think you need to measure things not influenced by recall bias," she said.

Recall bias, the tendency for memory to distort, riddled her miscarriage studies, Paigen said, and she never published her findings. She interviewed residents about their miscarriages mainly to prod the epidemiologists at the New York State Department of Health—which first raised the possibility of using miscarriage as an indicator of harm—to conduct more extensive analyses themselves. "I don't think I would have looked at miscarriage at all," she said. "It's embarrassing as a scientist to have to defend this. I did it with no money. I initially never intended it to be public. My purpose was to see if Love Canal people were totally crazy. I thought the health department would look at it more carefully." Indeed, she so tired of battling the health department over miscarriage, clouding her other findings, that at one point she conceded flat out that *their* studies, which relied on medical records rather than recall, had more validity. "I stopped talking about miscarriage, and I was hoping that would end it."

Even with her reservations about the miscarriage data, at the outset of our conversation, Paigen felt confident that Love Canal had led to increases in pregnancy loss. But after we revisited the old findings point by point, her perspective markedly changed. "At the time it seemed reasonable to me," she said, rightly noting that twenty-five years ago, scientists knew much less about the incidence of miscarriage and its causes than they do now. The next day, she e-mailed me a gracious note, writing that "you have gone a long way towards convincing me that miscarriage may not be a good indicator for toxic exposure."

I share Paigen's conviction that, as she once argued, the public does not require incontrovertible scientific proof before responding to a bomb threat, and it similarly should not require 95 percent certainty before taking action when confronted with hundreds of buried chemicals leaching into homes and a schoolyard. If my family lived at Love Canal and we had the wherewithal, I suspect I strongly would have advocated moving away. But the evidence that Love Canal increased miscarriages, at least knowing what I know today, would have had nothing to do with anything.

The Love Canal saga unfolds like a cinematic epic. From its hugely ambitious origins to the double-entendre name, the innocent young victims, the bungling by politicians and industry, the drawn-out drama of the residents, the discovery of deadly chemicals, the specious scientific studies, the lawsuits, the attention from the international media, and even the involvement of the White House, Love Canal had most every ingredient that makes Hollywood salivate. But Love Canal, which did become a made-for-television movie, lacked a crucial factor that helped propel *Erin Brockovich* and *A Civil Action* to the big screen: a cluster of a rare health problem. When a cluster of children who live within a few blocks of one another develop leukemia, it provides a powerful narrative. Miscarriage, the sentinel malady that helped transform Love Canal into an internationally followed soap opera, occurs often. Not only does this frequency significantly lessen the dramatic impact when a cluster surfaces, but it also makes the scientific mystery that much more difficult to unravel. "Can you use miscarriage as an index of environmental exposure?" Dorothy Warburton rhetorically asked me. "It's very, very tough to figure out whether environmental effects are real."

Simply consider how the researchers who studied health effects at Love Canal attempted to determine whether an increase in miscarriage had occurred. They first had to determine the normal rate of miscarriage, so they compared women either to their own previous pregnancy histories or to the old Warburton-Fraser data. Warburton and Fraser, who did their study by interviewing women between 1952 and 1962, found a miscarriage rate of 15 percent. As Wilcox's famous 1988 pee study (which relied on a sensitive human chorionic gonadotropin test to assess pregnancy) showed, 31 percent of women actually miscarry at implantation. In practice, pregnancy tests steadily have become more sensitive and diverse—including the introduction of ultrasounds done from inside the vagina—allowing more women to learn about miscarriages that in the

1950s may well have gone undetected. How did this bias the Love Canal population, which the best of the studies indicated had an overall miscarriage rate of about 22 percent? The result has no meaning. Comparing women to their own past pregnancies has less meaning still.

Warburton and her coworkers have studied a wide array of potential environmental causes of miscarriage—including caffeine, cigarettes, artificial sweeteners, marijuana, and cocaine—and have worked diligently to eliminate confounding variables that can distort conclusions. Their meticulous studies account for a woman's age and the number of previous miscarriages she has had, both of which can skew analyses. When possible, they have separated out chromosomally abnormal—and destined-to-fail—miscarriages from chromosomally normal ones. They have relied on staggering numbers of participants and samples: in one smoking study, they reported having interviewed 6,544 women who had miscarried and then successfully karyotyping 2,663 of the conceptuses. They rigorously attempted to match the women who miscarried to an equal numbers of controls who had similar ages, ethnicities, education, pregnancy histories, and socioeconomic backgrounds.

When I first spoke with Warburton in May 2001, I asked her what she thought of environmental causes of miscarriage. Her candid response stunned me. "I spent a lot of my life, unfortunately, trying to find the relationship between environmental factors and miscarriage with completely negative results," Warburton told me. "I don't think there's any strong evidence that environmental factors cause miscarriage."

A few years later, when we were discussing Love Canal, she made a similar point. "I've spent most of my life arguing against these isolated reports of increases of this and increases of that," she said. "It just goes on and on." Yet, a scientist to the core, she stressed that she kept an open mind. "We could miss things because we are so skeptical."

Using the Lexis Nexis database of newspapers, I found more than 150 stories worldwide that linked miscarriages to environmental and lifestyle causes between 1998 and 2003. Frequently based on new scientific studies, the reports, read together, create the horror-movie feeling of danger

lurking absolutely everywhere. Aside from the most famous alleged culprits—coffee, cigarettes, and illegal drugs—the stories warned that pregnant women should not swim in chlorinated pools; take anti-inflamma-
tory drugs like aspirin and ibuprofen; drink tap water; spray a common
weed killer; shower; use certain paints or some hair dryers, vacuum clean-
ers, and electric shavers that produce strong electromagnetic fields. Miscarriage clusters have occurred at a trailer park in Plaquemine, Louisiana
(near a Dow chemical plant), the Saltonstall office building in Boston,
the Shoalwater Bay Indian Reservation in Washington State, the USA Today
newsroom, the northern California public housing complex known as
Midway Village (near an old gas manufacturing plant), and in Pancevo,
Yugoslavia (NATO bombed a petrochemical plant and oil refinery during
the Balkan war). A Scottish paper warned about popular high-energy caffeine drinks, like Red Bull. In Canada, a report suggested that women
married to auto mechanics had a higher risk of miscarrying.

The many of the stories include the appropriate caveats from reproductive experts, who typically spot flaws in study design or flag other studies
that arrived at different conclusions, but I suspect that does little to mit-
igate the overwhelming sense of confusion and fear that these news reports create. Would that more of the journalists had first read a magnif-
icent survey of studies that tie environmental toxins to miscarriage
published in 2000 in the somewhat obscure Seminars in Reproductive Medicine. Cowritten by the ob-gyn Joseph Hill, then head of Harvard Medical
School's recurrent miscarriage clinic at Brigham and Women's Hospital,
the review analyzed twenty-five different potential causes. It also offered
something of a pocket guide to evaluate claims. Besides finding an increase in miscarriage rates in an exposed versus an unexposed group, a
study that purports to have found a dangerous environmental toxin ideally should also demonstrate increasing effects at higher doses of the
agent, a plausible biological mechanism for the effect, similar results in
animal experiments, and a threshold effect that delineates the exposure
or dose level at which harm occurs.

The paper includes a table that lists fifty-six known "teratogens,"
agents that can harm developing embryos and fetuses. Only one teratogen clearly caused a rise in miscarriages via an environmental contami-

nation: the ionizing radiation from atomic fallout after the U.S. bombing of Hiroshima and Nagasaki.

Mercury without question harms fetuses, but Hill and his coauthor Jennifer Gardella dismissed reports that female dentists and dental assistants miscarried more frequently because of exposure to mercury vapors from fillings. Lead also can cause prenatal harm—women in the early 1900s used lead pills as an abortifacient—but such use has become uncommon and regulations about exposure to it have tightened.

Hill and Gardella reported that no convincing evidence exists that environmental exposures to any of the following increase miscarriage risks: first-trimester diagnostic X-rays, air travel, ultrasound, electromagnetic fields, video displays (a famous 1988 study), aspartame, saccharin, chocolate, dioxin, pesticides, or hair dyes.

Similarly, they gave short shrift to concerns that a father's exposures to a teratogen could increase miscarriage rates. Soldiers exposed to Agent Orange or who served in Desert Storm, janitors, firemen, electricians, carpenters, and others exposed to toxins may well die themselves before their seminal fluid carries the teratogen to the mother or their sperm develops a chromosomal abnormality.

The many studies that have assessed the impact of cigarette smoking on miscarriage yielded conflicting results, in part because of the difficulty of separating its effects from that of alcohol. One massive study of more than 30,000 pregnant women that adjusted for alcohol use found only a significant increase in miscarriage in women who smoked more than two packs a day. Hill and Gardella, who lumped together studies involving a total of some 100,000 pregnant women, concluded that those who smoked between ten and twenty cigarettes a day became 1.1 times to 1.3 times more likely to miscarry. In other words, if an effect exists, it is modest.

Coffee, one of the world's most treasured stimulants, has received intense scrutiny from miscarriage researchers. Although studies have linked drinking more than three cups of coffee a day to miscarriage, Hill and Gardella note that in successful pregnancies, women often experience more nausea and decrease their coffee consumption. This phenomenon presents what scientists call a confounding variable, invalidating the findings about the three daily cups. When researchers dosed rodents with caffeine—either by injection or intubation—miscarriages and fetal deaths doubled, but Hill and Gardella noted that the dose used was the equivalent of a human drinking nearly a *gallon* of coffee a day.

Drinking alcohol during pregnancy can cause fetal alcohol syndrome, symptoms of which include low birth weight, neurological problems, learning disabilities, and facial anomalies. But a dozen recent alcohol-and-miscarriage studies have reached opposite conclusions. Again, people who drink heavily often smoke, do illegal drugs, and have poor diets, all factors that make it maddeningly difficult to separate out the impact of alcohol itself. Researchers also typically rely on women's self-reporting of alcohol consumption, and, logically enough, this method can lead to underreporting problems that further confuse the data. The largest study I found, involving more than 20,000 pregnant Danish women, discovered that women who reported having five or more glasses of beer, wine, or schnapps a week had more than three times as many miscarriages. But then the study had an overall miscarriage frequency of 1.8 percent, a number so out of sync with reality that it calls into question any supposed increase they found.

Warburton, her colleague Jennie Kline, and their coworkers published a paper in 1980 that reported a striking increase in miscarriage related to alcohol use: about 25 percent of women who drank twice a week or more had a pregnancy loss as compared to 14 percent of women who reported drinking less than that amount. But the researchers later divided the miscarriages by their chromosomal makeup, or karyotype; if alcohol played a role, the women who drank more should have had more chromosomally *normal* losses. No such distinction existed. Further complicating the matter, the investigation found the miscarriage-alcohol connection only in the patients who used public clinics and hospitals, not in the wealthier patients who received private care. "The conclusion is that it's very hard to make biological sense of the findings," Warburton told me. It is this type of scientific rigor that separates the Warburtons and Klines from many of their colleagues.

Chlorinated tap water, commonly thought of as the safest of all drinks, repeatedly has grabbed headlines for supposedly causing miscarriages. One widely publicized study in 1998 reported that researchers from the California Department of Health Services found that drinking a lot of cold tap water during the first trimester could, in some specific cases, nearly double the risk of miscarrying. The increased risk surfaced in 121 pregnant women out of 5,144 in the study who drank five or more daily glasses of cold tap water that had what the scientists considered high levels of trihalomethanes, a byproduct of chlorinated water. This group had a miscarriage rate of about 16 percent—twice as high as women who drank five or more glasses of cold tap water that had a low level of trihalomethanes. Aside from the fact that the researchers did not separate out chromosomally abnormal from normal miscarriages, these miscarriages represented a tiny fraction (2 percent) of the overall study population, a point the researchers stressed.

For two days in a row, page-one articles about the tap water study appeared in the *Los Angeles Times*, which broke the story after receiving leaked memos about the upcoming publication of the findings in a scientific journal. The stories' headlines would send shivers up any pregnant woman's spine. "New Worry for Pregnant Women," read one. Shanna Swan, the lead author of the study, told me that the coverage appalled her. "I'm a public health person," she said. "This put people in the terrible position of being very frightened and not having answers."

After a water official suggested that pregnant women boil tap water before drinking it, Swan and her coauthors noted that boiling might concentrate the trihalomethanes or send them into the air. Bottled water did not offer a solution, as it contains varying amounts of these chemicals. Although showering and swimming also can increase a person's exposure to trihalomethanes, the study did not find that those activities increased risks. Phew.

The L.A. *Times* follow-up coverage a few days later was even worse. "In the waiting room of the UCLA obstetrics and gynecology center, Melissa Jurist, 10 weeks' pregnant with her second child, fiddled nervously with a tissue Tuesday and wondered how best to make drinking water safe for her unborn baby." The story did quote a skeptical expert on prenatal exposure at the university's medical center, who "stressed that on the long list of environmental toxins harmful to unborn babies, tap water would be near the bottom."

Shanna Swan, now a researcher at the University of Missouri, Columbia, said she suspects that chlorinated water contains toxins that cause reproductive problems, but "they're unlikely to be trihalomethanes." She noted that the water treatment process creates about four hundred byproducts, making it extremely difficult to unscramble cause and effect. "We're in the course of learning about this," she said. "If it takes fifty years, we're maybe at the twenty-year point."

In keeping with Dorothy Warburton's counsel that too much skepticism also can mislead, a few environmental factors besides atomic bombs likely can cause miscarriage.

While the vast majority of bacterial and viral infections cause no harm to embryos or fetuses, a few pathogens may account for a small percentage of miscarriages, although their sporadic nature means they play no important role in recurrent loss. (They can lead to stillbirths, too, but that topic raises a range of issues unrelated to miscarriage.) A wide variety of mechanisms can lead to miscarriages. A mother's own symptoms, such as dangerously high temperatures or compromised immune systems, can harm an embryo or fetus. Infections can damage the placenta, the uterus, or lead to premature rupture of membranes. Some infectious agents can directly infect the embryo or fetus.

Scientists suspect that the bugs responsible for the following well-known diseases can cause miscarriages: rubella, syphilis, genital herpes, mumps, toxoplasmosis, malaria, and AIDS. Vaccines prevent rubella and mumps. Although no vaccines exist for genital herpes and toxoplasmosis (a disease mainly transmitted to humans by cats), humans develop immunity to these diseases after the first exposure, limiting the infection, so they likely play no role in miscarriages among woman who had these bugs before becoming pregnant. For sexually transmitted diseases such as syphilis, genital herpes, and AIDS, screening tests can help couples determine whether either partner has any of these infections and, in each case, drug treatment can help lower (or in the case of syphilis, eliminate) the risk of transmission between partners and babies.

Researchers have paid much attention to the possible links between miscarriage and an exotic-sounding list of bugs that includes *Listeria monocytogenes*, parvovirus B19, cytomegalovirus, *Ureaplasma urealyticum*, and the combined impact of the bacteria known as *Gardnerella vaginalis* and *Mycoplasma hominis*. *Listeria*, a bacterial infection spread by contaminated eggs, unpasteurized soft cheeses, and undercooked meats, has produced sound recommendation that pregnant women skip the raw egg in their Caesar salad dressings, the carpaccio at Italian restaurants, and the Brie and Camembert on cheese plates. Parvovirus, a rare infection, can cause fluid to build up in the fetus and lead to late miscarriages. Cytomegalovirus, a member of the herpes family, infects (but with few, if any, visible symptoms) more than half of the adults in the United States by the time they reach forty years old, and while it can cause harm to fetuses and people with damaged immune systems, it has no strong link to miscarriage. Several miscarriage studies have implicated *Ureaplasma urealyticum*, a parasite that lives in the genital tract of males and females and is so common that some scientists believe it has developed a symbiotic relationship with humans.

Gardnerella vaginalis and *Mycoplasma hominis* work together to cause bacterial vaginosis, an imbalance in the vaginal flora which results in a fishy-smelling discharge and premature rupture of membranes. Several studies have evaluated whether treating bacterial vaginosis can prevent late miscarriages, and such treatments have had mixed results. The most convincing, a double-blind, randomized, placebo-controlled study that involved nearly five hundred women in London reduced both late miscarriages (from 4 percent to 1 percent) and preterm deliveries (12 to 5 percent). The small number of women who had these serious problems in the study—late miscarriage totaled only twelve—has led to a call for still more studies before concluding that treatment helps. And some researchers stress that the studies simultaneously should treat male partners to prevent them from repeatedly reintroducing the infection.

In March 2003, I met a woman through an online miscarriage bulletin board who persuaded me that one water contaminant, nitrates, should receive a proper scientific study, which never has occurred, and rightly should concern the people who consume well water. (In the United States alone, 14 million homes rely on wells.) High levels of nitrates commonly enter wells from animal wastes on farms, fertilizer used on crops, or human sewage systems. When ingested, nitrates convert into nitrites, which modify hemoglobin such that it no longer can carry oxygen. In infants, this phenomenon leads to a life-threatening condition, blue baby syndrome. Because of this possibility, the EPA stipulates a maximum amount of nitrate that water can contain (no more than 10 milligrams per liter, or 0.0003 ounce per quart). A U.S. Geological Survey published in 1995 found that nearly one in ten household wells exceeded the standard.

The woman, who asked that I refer to her by her initials and her home state, C.S. from Oregon, had a harrowing pregnancy history. She first became pregnant at twenty-seven and, at her thirtieth week, developed the hallmark high blood pressure of preeclampsia. In September 1999, after five weeks of bed rest, C.S.'s blood pressure remained dangerously high, so her doctor admitted her to the hospital for treatment. Two days later, the drugs having failed to resolve her preeclampsia, the doctors induced her, but shortly after her water broke, they realized that the baby was in trouble and performed an emergency cesarean section.

The baby boy had a rare condition, vasa previa, in which the blood vessels of the umbilical cord grow in the wrong place. When the water breaks and labor begins, the delicate vessels can move into the birth canal ahead of the baby, leading to hemorrhage and, typically, its death. The doctors performed a blood transfusion and cardiopulmonary resuscitation on the boy whom C.S. had carried for thirty-five weeks, but he did not survive. "The emotional wounds did not heal for almost two years," C.S. wrote me. "Wrapped up in my grief, I was also afraid of not being able to have another baby. I'm not sure if this is a normal feeling in this kind of grief or if I had some premonition of what was to come."

In July 2000, C.S. became pregnant for the second time. An ultrasound at seven weeks showed an empty sac and no heartbeat. The doctor offered to send the distraught C.S. over to the nearby hospital for a higher-resolution ultrasound, but she and her husband had to catch an airplane flight to Minnesota and did not have time. "I cried all the way to Minnesota, and even that night in the hotel room," she told me. "We decided to hope for the best and wait and see. At this point, I wasn't willing to call it a miscarriage until I was actually bleeding." When she returned home the next week, another ultrasound had the same result as the first. She started to bleed heavily a few days later, and ended up in the emergency room for a D and C, in more pain than when she went into labor with her first pregnancy. "After this, the quest to become pregnant again became almost an obsession," C.S. said.

Depressed by each subsequent period, which she considered a "mini loss," in January 2001 she had an odd cycle, with intermittent light bleeding. A blood test bowled her over: she was pregnant again. But she quickly miscarried.

C.S. used home pregnancy tests every month, just in case. "I couldn't just let it be," she said. "I have an inquisitive and analytical nature, and letting it go is just not in my personality. It drove my husband crazy and drove a rift between us. He wouldn't talk, and I talked about it all the time."

C.S. enrolled in beauty school, and that summer learned she was pregnant again. She began having what she described as "mini panic attacks," worrying about the chemicals at the school and the cigarette smoke in the break room. She became particularly incensed by one pregnant woman at the school who smoked herself. Finally, she went over the edge when an instructor said, "If you don't calm down, you are going to cause yourself to have a miscarriage!" A grief counselor she met after losing her son suggested that she treat her panic attacks as though she were astride a startled horse—hang on and ride it out. "This helped me more than I can ever say," she remembered. "When dealing with grief and loss, nothing is familiar anymore. Half the time, I didn't even know myself." She soon had her third miscarriage.

C.S. asked her ob-gyn to do a thorough workup of her blood, but a series of tests did not reveal any problems. That November, she had a fourth miscarriage at her husband's fortieth birthday party. "I drank good beer and had a good time and tried to forget that we may never have a child," she said. "In my heart, I was scared."

A meeting with a reproductive endocrinologist led to a hysteroscopy that showed no abnormalities. But C.S. and her husband could not afford the other tests the doctor recommended. "I was disappointed and discouraged, and the toll on our marriage was reaching a critical point," she said. "We were making love only once a month when I said it was time. We barely had the heart for it." But their relationship began to improve when a client at work gave her a hot tub (another activity that researchers have tried mightily to tie to miscarriage with little success). "I felt like we'd won the lottery," C.S. said. "Our marriage desperately needed a break and some fun."

They stopped their intensive efforts to become pregnant, which happened again in September 2002 with yet another early miscarriage. "This lit a fire under me," she said, adding that she had a new job and now could afford more tests. "I went into overdrive mode to have a baby." Much to her disappointment, a battery of new tests revealed nothing. "I was wishing there was something medically wrong with me so we could treat *something*." To increase their chances of becoming pregnant yet again, they opted for Clomid and intrauterine sperm injections. It worked, but she quickly miscarried in October. "I was starting to get used to it," C.S. said. "I guess you just have to develop a hard heart or go completely insane." The same thing happened in November.

Then they had a kitchen problem that she believes altered their fate. Because of water damage, their kitchen needed extensive remodeling, so they moved to a hotel for the Christmas holidays. Without medical help, they conceived during their relocation, and at six weeks had a heartbeat, the first since their son. But the sac had not grown. The specialist they saw, who prided himself on being able to tell which ones would make it, said she had a 75 percent chance of miscarrying, predicting that each week, the heartbeat would become slower until the baby died.

C.S. returned to her regular obstetrician and had another ultrasound the next week. The heartbeat was strong, and the growth looked normal.

Curious as to why, after seven miscarriages, this baby had made it further than all of the rest, C.S. thought long and hard about what she had done differently. Their property has a well, and her mother repeatedly had suggested that the water in it might be the key to the string of miscarriages. This time, when she conceived they had stopped drinking from the well because of their kitchen overhaul, and they ate all of their meals at restaurants. She also recalled that when she became pregnant the first time they had a reverse osmosis water purification system for drinking water, which they stopped using after they purchased a refrigerator with a cold water dispenser—and no filter. She typed into an Internet search engine "well water miscarriage" and found page after page about nitrates in well water, which particularly pose problems in farming communities, like hers, which liberally use manure for fertilizers. She also until recently had raised chickens, which further could elevate nitrate levels through their feces. C.S. decided she would drink only bottled, purified water for the duration of the pregnancy.

In September 2003, she gave birth to a healthy, seven-pound, twelve-ounce boy.

A 1961 study implicated nitrates as a possible cause of human miscarriage, as have several animal studies. But no other human studies on the topic appeared in the scientific literature for thirty-five years, when *Morbidity and Mortality Weekly Report*, a widely read bulletin put out by the U.S. Centers for Disease Control and Prevention, published an investigation of a miscarriage cluster.

Between May 1991 and December 1992, a thirty-five-year-old woman in LaGrange County, Indiana, had four early miscarriages, which caught the attention of the local health department by happenstance. William Grant, a LaGrange County Health Department biologist, explained to me that a woman phoned who had found high nitrate levels in her well and wanted him to stop by. "As we were talking about her situation, she happened to mention that the lady up the road had had four consecutive miscarriages," said Grant. "I thought that was curious." During his subsequent investigation, Grant discovered that two other women in the vicinity recently had miscarried. A well at a nearby hog farm in 1989 had a nitrate contamination of greater than fifty milligrams per liter—five times the EPA standard, so Grant and his coworkers measured each woman's well for possible contaminants. They found only one, nitrate, and it was roughly twice as high as the standard in each well. The wells of five other neighbors who recently had given birth were checked, too, and all registered acceptable.

The health department soon learned of a fourth intriguing case, a thirty-five-year-old woman who had five children and then two back-to-back early miscarriages. Her well, which she had not used for four of her five pregnancies, had a nitrate level nearly three times higher than the standard.

All four women, the researchers noted, switched to bottled water or reverse-osmosis systems and later gave birth to healthy babies.

These few cases hardly constitute proof of causation. But given the proven dangers of nitrates to infants, I think that checking well water for levels of nitrates (which fluctuate seasonally) falls squarely into the category of common sense—regardless of whether someone in the house is trying to conceive.

Science is provisional. What appears real today may, based on new evidence, seem naïve tomorrow. Future research may discover irrefutable evidence that something in the environment causes miscarriages and that science overlooked, ignored, or wrongly judged this teratogen. A laboratory mishap that occurred in 1998 illustrates how a chance discovery can lead the most confirmed skeptics to do a double take.

In August of that year, the geneticist Patricia Hunt noticed a bizarre change in the eggs of the female mice she studies. For some inexplicable reason, the chromosomes in 40 percent of the eggs looked abnormal— a wild jump from the 1 percent to 2 percent abnormality her lab typically observes. Something seemed to have gone terribly wrong with meiosis, the process that separates chromosomes during reproduction so that when egg and sperm come together they each contribute half the genetic material to an embryo. Hunt, whose lab at Case Western Reserve University in Cleveland specializes in problems with meiosis and miscarriage, asked her technicians to redo the study twice, yielding the same baffling results each time.

The first clue came that fall, when Hunt noticed that her mouse cages, made of a plastic called polycarbonate, appeared to be melting. She found that an assistant had mistakenly washed the cages with a highly alkaline detergent. "He was a temporary worker who made a lasting impression," Hunt joked. Hunt, her husband and coworker Terry Hassold, and their colleagues, eventually pinned the meiotic abnormalities on a chemical called bisphenol A (BPA), which had leached from the damaged plastic cages. Although several labs have shown that BPA, a compound widely used in plastics manufacturing, can disrupt the reproductive system of rodents, none had previously shown an effect on meiosis.

The detective work, which they published in 2003, thrust Hunt's lab into the middle of the controversial field of endocrine disruptors. Some researchers and environmentalists have argued that low levels of certain synthetic chemicals in the environment cause reproductive problems in wildlife, and perhaps in humans. BPA, which weakly mimics the effects of estrogen, has been among the suspects.

I spoke with researchers from many disciplines about the finding, including Texas A&M's Stephen Safe, a leading skeptic of evidence linking endocrine disruptors to health problems, who said he found the data "very interesting." Leading proponents of BPA's harmful effects predictably had stronger words: "I look at this as a watershed paper," said the reproductive biologist Frederick vom Saal of the University of Missouri, Columbia, whose lab has published several studies about BPA's impact on mouse reproductive development.

Hunt and her coworkers first noticed problems when they took a routine "snapshot" of the meiotic process in their mice. They found that 40 percent of the mouse eggs failed to assemble their chromosomes neatly on the spindle apparatus, a step that must occur for separation to take place properly. They also found abnormal numbers of chromosomes, the aberration called aneuploidy, in about 12 percent of the eggs. "When I read that I said, Zowee, that's really out of sight," said John Eppig, a reproduction biologist at Jackson Laboratory in Bar Harbor, Maine.

Once they suspected BPA, Hunt's lab recreated the accident. They intentionally damaged polycarbonate cages and water bottles with detergent, and compared the mice in those cages to animals kept in undamaged cages with glass bottles. They found the same levels of meiotic error in the damaged cages. They then showed that BPA was the culprit by adding the chemical to mouse water; it caused chromosomal problems, though not as severe.

The results turned even the head of Dorothy Warburton. "It's probably the only convincing demonstration of an environmental effect on the frequency of aneuploidy," she told me. "It's a little scary."

Although Hunt noted that no evidence clearly links BPA to human miscarriage, she thinks the question deserves serious investigation because the compound is so widely used: Plastics made from it are in baby bottles, the liners of food cans, dental sealants, and many other common products. Dorothy Warburton told me that she planned to measure BPA levels in a new, large miscarriage study she launched in 2003.

My father's mother, a poor woman from Yemen, grew to loathe her husband, whom she wed in an arranged marriage. Yona gave birth to ten children, five of whom died young from disease. At forty-two, she became pregnant with my father, the last of the lot, and she desperately wished to miscarry. Thinking no one would be the wiser, she repeatedly stood on a chair and jumped to the ground. My aunt would love telling this story to tease my father, who did not suffer any obvious damage from the early assaults.

Fetuses are more rugged than we think. That's not to suggest that they benefit from having their mothers repeatedly jump from a chair—or from exposure to bisphenol A, nitrates, dioxin, cigarette smoke, benzene, cocaine, pesticides, and dozens of other toxins. But what the research has shown to date does not so much illuminate the dangers that these environmental hazards present to embryos and fetuses as it highlights how remarkable an environment the female body provides for babies. The uterus, amniotic sac, and the placenta marvelously work together to prevent harm, and, although the system has its weaknesses, I doubt that the most creative minds on the planet could devise a better one.

Miscarriages, as far as science can now determine, rarely occur because of what a woman eats or drinks, where she lives and works, or what air she breathes. More than half of all miscarriages have abnormal chromosomes, mainly because the mother's eggs do not properly execute meiosis. Other than BPA in mice and radiation exposure, I have seen no data that suggest an environmental force can mess with meiosis. For the other half of miscarriages that have normal chromosomes, science has arrived at a few clear-cut causes. As for the rest, the jury remains out, especially when it comes to the environment and lifestyle. And until research proves otherwise, this lack of evidence should offer some comfort to the many women who miscarry and blame themselves.

10

EXPERT CARE

IN ONE OF THE MOST PECULIAR MISCARRIAGE STUDIES EVER published, researchers in Oslo in 1984 reported that what they called "tender-loving care" had a dramatic impact on pregnant women who had a history of repeatedly miscarrying. Hard-core biomedical researchers typically blanch when confronted with such soft, touchy-feely findings. But the researchers who ran this study, Babill and Sverre Stray-Pedersen, a husband-and-wife research team who worked in the obstetrics and gynecology department of the University of Oslo, had hard-core credentials. Between them they studied infections and miscarriage, problems with amniotic fluid, chromosomal abnormalities of sperm, and osmosis in cellular membranes. The Stray-Pedersens found that out of a group of sixty-one pregnant women, 86 percent given tender-loving care, or TLC, carried to term, while the success rate plummeted to 33 percent in the group that received no specific treatment.

The nitty-gritty details of this study give it more weight. Over nine years, the researchers followed 195 women who came to the National Hospital in Oslo because they had at least three consecutive miscarriages. In all, the women, some of whom had had as many as thirteen losses, had a total of 773 clinically verified miscarriages. The researchers did a thorough diagnostic workup of these women and their partners, and discovered abnormalities that might have a link to miscarriage in 110 couples. They then aggressively treated these women for their specific problems, surgically correcting uterine anomalies, removing fibroids, performing cerclage on those deemed to have incompetent cervixes, injecting human chorionic gonadotropin for luteal phase deficiency, and giving drugs to clear Ureaplasma urealyticum and Toxoplasma gondii infections. In the eighty-five couples who had no detected abnormalities, sixty-one conceived, leading to the follow-up study of tender-loving care.

While twenty-four women did not receive any unusual care and visited their local prenatal clinics for checkups, the thirty-seven women in the TLC group visited the Stray-Pedersens and had weekly medical exams and "optimal psychological support." TLC also consisted of advising these women to avoid heavy work and travel, as well as bed rest during the two-week gestational period at which they had previously miscarried.

Miscarriage researchers far and wide noted the striking difference in the two groups—86 percent versus 33 percent—because it called into question every study that claimed to have had success with an intervention. If psychological support and weekly medical exams truly could influence whether a woman carried to term, then those forces might have confounded the success rates for progesterone, lymphocyte immune therapy, or even a surgery.

The Stray-Pedersens' tender-loving care study certainly had its methodological weaknesses, especially because the researchers did not divide the participants randomly into a treated and a control group (women who received TLC simply lived closer to the National Hospital). But seven years later, a more carefully controlled study published by New Zealand investigators presented more evidence that TLC had spectacular powers. At a recurrent miscarriage clinic in Auckland, Hilary Liddell, Neil Pattison, and Angi Zanderigo compared forty-two women in a group treated with "formal supportive care" to ten women randomly assigned to a control group who received standard care from a gynecological clinic. Women in both groups underwent identical exams—including hysterosalpingo-grams that X-rayed the uterus and fallopian tubes, as well as blood analyses for everything from infections to antiphospholipid antibodies—and all had no identified problems. Women in each group had an average of four previous miscarriages and were similar in age.

The treated group attended a physiotherapy class each week at which they learned relaxation skills. They also received a "relaxation tape," which the researchers asked them to use each day. "An appropriately decorated room was established in a hospital ward for the women if they wished to come into hospital, for example at the times of threatened miscarriage, or at the anniversary gestation of previous losses," the investigators explained. After the end of the first trimester—or past the gestation point from her most recent miscarriage—each woman saw her own practitioner, though most also stayed in contact with the miscarriage clinic. At the study's end, the Auckland group amazingly had identical results to the Stray-Pedersens' study: 86 percent in the treated group went to term, while the success dropped to 33 percent in the control group.

The researchers concluded that the significant difference between the groups "could well be due to the therapeutic effect of formal emotional support in early pregnancy." They further emphasized that repeatedly miscarrying creates a "very marked stress reaction" the next time a woman becomes pregnant:

> Observation shows that this stress reaction is characterized by general tension, weeping, fear of going to the toilet or of examining underwear in case of finding bleeding, checking continuously for continuance of pregnancy symptoms, extreme anxiety over any abdominal pain, discharge or change in symptoms, avoidance of other pregnant women or discussing the pregnancy with anyone including husbands, panic attack at the gestation of previous miscarriages as well as general despondence and assumption that "it will happen again."

As I read this last sentence to my wife, Shannon, she started yelling "yes!" repeatedly.

I see the limits of these two studies, both of which involved relatively small numbers of patients. Like scientists, I also squirm when confronted by psychobabbly hypotheses. If the cheesy wallpaper and motel art that clinics favor significantly affects whether a woman miscarries, a few good interior decorators could substantially alleviate a lot of misery and despair. And I bristle at the notion, as does Shannon, that stress triggered her four miscarriages, which one know-nothing implied after Ryan's birth, clapping me on the back, and saying, "Well, you finally relaxed." I do not know what, if anything, markedly changed in the way that either Shannon or I responded to that surprise pregnancy; she did not listen to relaxation tapes, and the grieving she did on the anniversaries of previous miscarriages was sporadic and unplanned.

Yet after I began to spend time at a few of the world's leading clinics for recurrent miscarriage, my reservations about these findings eased, and, eventually, they disappeared. Many a time as I sat and watched people visit a miscarriage clinic, with doctors and nurses listening to couples tell their sad histories and discuss their options, I thought to myself, They are lucky to have found expert care—care that Shannon and I never even knew existed. And the remarkable sentence that led Shannon to yell "yes!" powerfully reveals to me not what women go through who miscarry—I knew that up close—but, instead, the depth of insight that clinicians who work in this field can acquire.

Expert care matters, and the tender-loving aspect of it ultimately provides just one of many components that I am convinced help people carry to term. More important still, I believe that expert care helps people come to terms with their reproductive possibilities and limitations, regardless of whether they eventually carry to term. Yet miscarriage is one of those oddities in medicine: a common condition that has few true specialists. Surf the Internet to find departments of obstetrics and gynecology at universities with medical schools, which typically offer the best care across the board. If a program mentions miscarriage, it usually appears under the heading "reproductive endocrinology" or "infertility." Miscarriage is a sub-subspecialty. No one offers a degree in miscarriage-ology. There is no *Journal of Miscarriage*, no Society of Miscarriage Medicine that holds an annual meeting, and no formal assessment of the miscarriage care that does exist (the U.S. Congress, in contrast, in 1992 passed a law that *requires* fertility clinics that use assisted reproductive technologies to report their annual success rates). So it remains a huge challenge for miscarriage patients to find clinicians who know the latest research, provide proper evaluations, carefully prescribe interventions, and, yes, offer true TLC.

Just as scientific research can never prove that love exists, I suspect it can never arrive at rock-solid evidence that expert care prevents miscarriages or helps people come to terms with their reproductive fate. But as one researcher said to me, If you witness a talking dog, you do not need a control group to believe it. In three different recurrent miscarriage clinics around the world, I have seen the equivalent of a talking dog.

As I clomped through the Boston snow for my first visit to a clinic that specializes in miscarriage, I passed what once was called the Lying-In Hospital and then entered the former Free Hospital for Women, places where Arthur Hertig and John Rock a half century earlier conducted their pioneering egg hunt and captured the most detailed snapshots ever taken of early embryos traveling from tube to womb. I then entered the Fearing Research Laboratory, which in the Hertig-and-Rock era existed across town and served as the headquarters for Olive and George Smith's ill-fated studies of diethylstilbestrol. Winding through a few hallways I came to the office of Danny Schust, head of the recurrent miscarriage clinic at what today is known as Harvard Medical School's Brigham and Women's Hospital.

Schust, then thirty-eight, had become head of the clinic the year before when its longtime director, Joseph Hill, left for private practice. Schust had spent a decade doing basic research on the immune system and pregnancy but had not conducted any clinical studies yet of recurrent miscarriage. Still, he was well versed in the scientific literature and had just cowritten a superb overview of implantation that appeared in the *New England Journal of Medicine*. He also had a readily apparent kindness and a wry honesty. Shortly after we met, he said, "Women in general tolerate these procedures that we would never tolerate" — "we" meaning men. Women endure hysteroscopies, hysterosalpingograms, endometrial biopsies, intrauterine insemination, ovarian stimulation, and egg retrieval. "Ask men for a semen analysis, and it takes six months," he said. "It's an amazing thing."

Many private hospitals and infertility clinics in the United States have miscarriage specialists. Brigham and Women's remains the only non-profit I know of in the country that has a full-fledged recurrent miscarriage clinic. In the United Kingdom, recurrent miscarriage clinics exist in London, Liverpool, and Leeds. Canada has miscarriage clinics in Vancouver and Toronto. Australia's Royal Women's Hospital near Melbourne has one, as does neighboring New Zealand's National Women's Hospital in Auckland. An Internet search also turned up miscarriage clinics based at public hospitals in India, Ireland, Qatar, Israel, the United Arab Emirates, and Kuwait.

Before Joe Hill left, I spoke with him at some length about the economic disincentives to running a miscarriage clinic. "Ob-gyn is largely procedure-based," said Hill. "The differential of what can be made for procedures versus office consultations is two to three times. And people don't want to take the time to deal with these patients. This is very labor-intensive and reimbursement is largely lacking."

Other, noneconomic forces similarly dissuade physicians from specializing in miscarriage. "They're frustrating," Schust told me. "And it's a rapidly evolving, pseudoscience field, which is depressing."

The clinic at Brigham and Women's sees patients who have had at least two miscarriages, and the majority, Schust said, end up carrying to term. Like most every clinician I met who specialized in miscarriage, he liked the work because he liked the patients. To make this point, he compared the typical miscarriage patient to the women he met while working as a fellow in an infertility clinic. "We had a bunch of very empowered women who had waited a long time to try and have kids," he explained. "Throughout their lives they'd had success in everything they tried. They were trying to do something that they thought was a God-given right, and they were mad as hell." Miscarriage patients typically do not have as much anger, he said, adding that they reminded him of patients receiving treatment for cancer. "They're a little bit desperate because they want to do something, and, unfortunately, a lot of physicians are willing to test things on them," said Schust. "I learn a huge amount from them about the human spirit and how people endure." He noted, too, that he likes working with this population because most who become pregnant again will carry to term: several recurrent miscarriage clinics have reported that more than two-thirds of pregnant women with a history of three miscarriages will carry to term.

The Brigham and Women's clinic sees about 150 new patients each year, and Schust says he treats only about half of them. "I've tried to limit interventions to things that have good data," he said. For one-third of the patients, Schust does not even arrive at a diagnosis of any specific problem.

I shadowed Schust at his clinic for a day, and some patients allowed me to observe their consultations. I have no idea whether the medical care they received ultimately helped them realize their dreams, and I had no intention of formally evaluating this clinic or any other. Rather, I wanted a sense of how each clinic operated—the people who came in, the questions they asked, and how Schust and the other miscarriage professionals I observed dealt with their typically distraught patients, each of whom had a unique, raw history, as well as a different host of problems and desires. And, in the end, I hope that an up-close look at the clinicians who specialize in miscarriage will give people who need help a better sense of what expert care looks like.

When Danny Schust's first patient entered the consultation room clutching a red-covered Holy Bible, it created a confessional atmosphere, which became more pronounced as she discussed her hopes and fears. The thirty-year-old woman, a veteran of the clinic, had two children and seven documented miscarriages, though she thought she had had a total of twelve. She had a uterine septum, earlier removed, and a blood-clotting disorder. Schust gently told her that he could not help her.

Recently remarried, the woman wanted more children. Her husband, she unabashedly explained, had yet to have his sperm examined. "He came here and tried to do a sample, but he couldn't," she explained.

Painful endometriosis had led her to take Lupron, a drug that blocks the effects of gonadotropin-releasing hormone, and, as a result, prevented her from ovulating. Given her desire to have more children and her complaints of knee pains and muscle weakness, known side effects of Lupron, Schust logically suggested that she stop the drug. "I'd probably recommend you go straight to IVF," Schust said.

When women who repeatedly miscarry consider in vitro fertilization, they frequently find themselves confronted with a possibility that borders on the absurd: the procedure, which often transfers multiple embryos with the hope that one will take, may lead them to have *more* children than they want. This woman worried mightily about this scenario. "I come from an incredibly religious family," she said, stressing that they would not approve of her going through selective reduction. "If I were to get pregnant with four of these, I'd be put through hell by these guys," she said. Schust assured her that they probably would transfer only two, which led her to question whether those two embryos could split into multiples. "We can't control that," he said. She fiddled with her Bible.

His second patient that day had a complicated history, too: one child, two "therapeutic terminations"—the euphemism for abortions because of bad amniocentesis or ultrasound results—and three early miscarriages. Originally from Africa, she had had a fibroid removed, and during the last two menstrual cycles, had tried Clomid with artificial insemination. She, too, had deep reservations about multiples. "Two is fine," she said. "Three I don't need." She turned to me, plaintively. "I need one more," she said. "I have a boy who is eight. I *planned one more.*"

A couple from a Slavic country was next. The thirty-eight-year-old woman, who had two daughters, subsequently had four miscarriages and one termination after amniocentesis revealed a trisomy, three copies of one chromosome. The chromosomal abnormality, coupled with a karyotype of one miscarriage that also showed a trisomy, led the couple to wonder whether they had something fundamentally wrong with their genes. A test of their chromosomes discovered no underlying problem. Schust assured them, to their obvious disbelief, that many couples conceive two trisomic babies, and most likely it reflects nothing more than a run of bad luck.

"There's a lot of controversy about recurrent miscarriage," explained Schust. "One reason is because it's the final outcome of a lot of different disorders. People with recurrent miscarriage also tend to do really well. Even with three or four or five. If you become pregnant again, you're likely to have another child."

"Really?" the woman said, clearly astonished.

As he repeatedly did during the day, Schust carefully and accurately walked them through the available tests, from the least to the most invasive, tutoring them along the way about the various interventions, including unproven ones, now available. Schust advised starting slowly by testing her blood and doing a hysterosalpingogram to make sure her uterus and tubes had no obstructions.

"Do you ever have to tell someone, 'Don't keep trying to have children'?" the woman asked.

"It becomes a question of how many times you want to get on the roller coaster," Schust replied. "Some people quit after two times, some after ten. It's a hard decision. It's horrible."

After they left, Schust filled in a few notes on their charts. "My guess is they'll be fine," he told me.

A husband and wife arrived next, requesting that Schust write a referral letter to Alan Beer, the private practitioner who long advocated lymphocyte immune therapy and other experimental treatments that aim to tame the mother's immune reaction to her offspring. "I'm killing off my babies," the woman said.

After having one child, the woman had eight losses. Her husband confided that when they had seen Joe Hill in the past, he had strong criticisms of Beer. Schust took a more diplomatic approach, suggesting that some of the treatments Beer uses might help some people. "Maybe you're the person who will benefit from it," said Schust. "I don't know." Schust gave the couple a long, sympathetic look. "And I don't think he knows." The husband turned to me and whispered under his breath, "I told her I'm never going to get her pregnant again."

When Schust's patients have a healthy, uncomplicated pregnancy, they leave his care and return to their regular obstetricians to help them all the way through to labor and delivery. "It's always a good thing when I say good-bye," said Schust.

Mary Stephenson's recurrent miscarriage clinic was in a large, faded yellow building near downtown Vancouver which once served as a hospital for Canadian veterans returning from World War II. The former veterans hospital served as a perfect backdrop, as many of the women who attend the clinic have the demeanor of war veterans: they see the world through a different lens and have difficulty explaining it to those who never have experienced this tragic, frightening place that no imagination could accurately render. To a person, they see the limited ability they have to control their fate, and for some, it has religious overtones, confirming or resurrecting their faith in a supreme power. For others, it remains more existentialist than divine. This is my hand, they say, and I will play it the best I can. Either way, these women, just as I had seen in my own wife, develop a sad wisdom.

As I did at Brigham and Women's, I observed Stephenson working with patients, but one day I also met privately with a half dozen people who had seen her for several years. Stephenson's buoyant, theatrical personality counters the anguish and anxiety of her patients. Sitting in her office cubicle, she lifted a file folder stuffed with papers, and explained to me how, as a medical student, she became interested in miscarriage when she did her rotation with infertility patients. "One of the doctors gave me a file like this, a typical infertility file," said Stephenson, who often telegraphs her reactions with a high-cocked brow, a mirthful smile, a squinted eye, or pursed lips. "So many of these patients had no answers. I just got so fascinated by it. It's so uncharted. It's like a whole new world."

Stephenson and her head nurse, Edwina Houlihan, selected the patients they thought I should meet. When journalists come knocking, many clinicians, often under the advice of an institution's public relations department, select patients who have similar, boosterish narratives that goes something like this: distraught patient, clever doctor makes tricky diagnosis, resourceful clinic provides cutting-edge treatment, treatment works, patient jumps and clicks heels. Stephenson and Houlihan did nothing of the sort. Instead, they introduced me to what I came to see as their clinic family, the patients they have worked with for years, who refer to Mary by her first name and drop by with their kids to catch up with Edwina. That day I met Mary Skarsgard, who after eight miscarriages and a corrected septate uterus had been thrilled to give birth to Christopher Lloyd, even though he had died at thirty-two-weeks gestation. They asked Marian Anderson if she would speak with me about the four miscarriages she had between her two sons, during which she was diagnosed with luteal phase deficiency and antiphospholipid syndrome. No one knows which, if any, of her extensive treatments helped her carry to term. The others I met, some of whom still desperately wanted children, had similarly illustrative, untidy reproductive and personal histories, and a few had decidedly unclear outcomes.

I first walked over to a wing of the attached hospital and visited Janet and her husband, Dennis, in a patient lounge. Janet, then thirty-two weeks pregnant, had moved into the hospital three weeks earlier when a routine prenatal exam found that her cervix had begun to dilate and funnel, signs of labor. Although bed rest never has formally proven itself as an effective way to prevent preterm labor, I soon understood why Janet, thirty-five, and Dennis, thirty-three, had no qualms about trading the comforts of home for several weeks of privacy deprivation, hospital food, and relentless monitoring of bodily functions.

After four miscarriages, Janet began seeing Stephenson in October 1998. "Mary said, 'Before we go anywhere, let's research the problem, let's figure it out,'" remembered Janet, who sat in a wheelchair. "It was reassuring." Dennis said he did not know what to think, but, in fine XY form, was confident that their problem was "easy to fix somehow." A hysteroscopy determined that Janet had a single, "horned" uterus, but Stephenson saw no need to operate. (This müllerian anomaly has a strong association with preterm labor.) When she failed to become pregnant in 1999, Janet went on Clomid and quickly became pregnant—and just as quickly miscarried. She cracked open her journal from that time, and read me a sentence. "I truly do not know where to turn," it said. She had another early miscarriage in 2000, bringing her total to six. "It was just heart-wrenching for my mom, because she couldn't have children," said Janet, who was adopted.

An endometrial biopsy suggested a luteal phase defect, so Janet began taking progesterone. Although she earlier had tested negative for antiphospholipid syndrome, a reevaluation discovered that she had turned strongly positive for one type of the antibodies that causes the condition. She began heparin injections and baby aspirin each day. A pregnancy that began in December 2000, aside from painful cramping, appeared to progress well through the first trimester. "We thought we were at the magic twelve weeks," said Dennis. But an ultrasound showed an increased thickening around the neck, a marker of Down syndrome. The baby girl also had a massive heart defect. Stephenson, too, became emotional about the tragic situation. "Janet, this looked so good, I wasn't anticipating anything," she told her. They terminated the pregnancy, which indeed had trisomy 21, at twenty-one weeks. "That ripped both of us to death," said Janet.

"We said, That's it, this is crazy, this is stupid, it's killing us," remembered Dennis. "There's more to life than having a child." They still keep the baby's ashes in a little bag in their dresser.

They pursued adoption, and leads in South America raised their hopes, until they ran into formidable legal issues. Janet went back on Clomid, heparin, aspirin, and progesterone and, in the fall of 2001, became pregnant for the eighth time. "You say you're going to stop, but it looms in your heart," said Janet. An ultrasound could not find a heartbeat. "Mary was so dumbfounded," said Janet. For the first time, they had a karyotype of a miscarriage, and it was chromosomally normal. "We said to ourselves, This is it," said Dennis.

In the spring of 2002, with no medical interventions and no planning, Janet became pregnant for the ninth time and had an early loss. "That was reckless living," said Janet. Miscarriage, especially after nine of them, can completely redefine how people view the process of making babies.

An adoption agency phoned with a lead. It would cost $30,000, and Janet and Dennis would have to meet with the birth mother at a Los Angeles hotel first. They made the trip, checking into a hotel room, with the woman in an adjacent room. At the last moment, Janet decided to pull the plug. "There were just too many variables to deal with," said Janet. "She had had four miscarriages and was four months along. As a woman who had had miscarriages, I couldn't cross that boundary."

They returned to Stephenson, who said, for the sake of Janet's health, she would help them only one more time, and they had to conceive and deliver before she turned thirty-six. Janet became pregnant a few months later and began having ultrasounds weekly, requesting that the scanner look for every organ in the body at each visit. "You don't take anything for granted," Janet said. Stephenson recalled that Janet for the first time had intense morning sickness, too, a sign of a healthy pregnancy. "She was so happy to be vomiting," Stephenson told me.

Before I left, Janet told me that the day before, thirty-two weeks into this pregnancy, she had, for the first time, felt relaxed and confident that all would work out well. (It did. A month later, Janet gave birth to a healthy baby boy.)

Back at the miscarriage clinic, I met with Katie, forty-five, and her husband, David, forty-one. Katie had two children from her first marriage, but then with David had three miscarriages, one of which had an abnormal karyotype, which led them six years ago to seek help from Stephenson. Katie also started to attend a support group at the clinic, which did not work well. "I felt ostracized by the other women, who thought, You already have two kids," said Katie.

Blood tests did not uncover any abnormalities, and Stephenson suggested that they not bother with a battery of tests. Katie became pregnant, but had another early miscarriage, which also had an abnormal karyotype. "Finding out what the reason was for the miscarriages made it easier to deal with—understanding that it wasn't compatible with life and that we had done everything we could do," said Katie. The repeated abnormal karyotypes also provided evidence that, in all likelihood, Katie did not have any fundamental, underlying problem.

She started taking baby aspirin, and the next year, in 1999, Katie gave birth to a healthy baby girl. Like many couples who attend the clinic, Katie and David chose Mary as a middle name. "I do believe if I hadn't been with Dr. Stephenson, we wouldn't have her," said Katie.

Katie had two more early miscarriages in 2000, both of which had abnormal karyotypes. The next year, Katie again miscarried twice. Only one of these miscarriages yielded a specimen for karyotyping, which—for the fifth time—proved chromosomally abnormal. "If she went elsewhere and didn't have the chromosomes analyzed, they would have had her on the whole works," Stephenson told me.

Katie spoke frankly with me about the oddity of a forty-five-year-old woman with three kids seeking help from a recurrent miscarriage clinic to have a fourth. She and David do not have an extended family, and her older children from her previous marriage have not grown up with their daughter. "We want her to have a sibling," said Katie. "And I have this need inside of me to have another child. I can't seem to knock it out." Even though she was at the "end of the age range," she continued to ovulate and her level of follicle-stimulating hormone had spiked, an indicator of the onset of menopause. "We still consider there's hope," said Katie. "If Dr. Stephenson didn't think it was worth it, I'd have to let go of this dream."

She draped her arms around her daughter, who had been shuttling in and out of the room with her father as we spoke. "Mary has the compassion and the medical expertise that make patients feel comfortable," said Katie. "And she's not sugarcoating anything. She was skeptical with this one all along." She gave her daughter a squeeze. "Mary gives us hope for a new life, and we're still crazy enough to keep on trying."

Stephenson invited me to watch her meet with one of the four hundred new patients she sees each year. The twenty-nine-year-old woman had miscarried only twice and had no known problem. "I want poopy diapers," the woman said. "I want screaming kids." Stephenson, a green rubber thimble on one finger, paged through a flip chart for the woman and her husband, slowly explaining the various causes and interventions of miscarriage. "I feel very comfortable saying just try again and I'll follow you closely," Stephenson concluded. "I'll see you soon with a positive pregnancy."

I thought the woman might jump across the table and kiss Stephenson. "I prayed last night that you would say, You're fine, get out of here, don't waste my time," she said.

"Well, you're not wasting my time," said Stephenson.

The woman warned Stephenson that when and if she did become pregnant, she might become a nuisance. "I'll be calling every day," she said. "And I hope I can't find you in the phone book, 'cause I'll hunt you down at home." Stephenson pursed her lips and lifted her eyebrows into a smile, as if to say, You'll be fine.

I asked Stephenson, who in February 2004 planned to leave Vancouver and start a new clinic based at the University of Chicago, what she thought of the power of tender-loving care. "I hate that phrase," she said. But she thought the clinic she ran did offer something unquantifiable that helped women, some way, somehow, carry to term. "It's about validation and control," Stephenson said. "It's OK to want to phone a nurse every day."

On April 27, 1938, four royal horse guardsmen at Buckingham Palace lured a fourteen-year-old girl into their barracks by claiming to have a horse with a green tail in their stables. The men gang-raped her. A month later, the girl's parents took her to the doctor for a pregnancy test, which proved positive. Her physician refused to perform an abortion, arguing that her child might be the future prime minister of England and that "girls always lead men on." When apprised of the situation, Aleck William Bourne, a prominent London obstetrician at St. Mary's Hospital —where Alexander Fleming ten years earlier had discovered penicillin— agreed to meet with the girl. After observing her for a few days, he concluded that giving birth could cause "injury to her mind" that might lead to "life-long neuroses which in turn can and does produce secondary organic disease."

Bourne performed the abortion, and that evening, the police—possibly tipped off by Bourne himself, who belonged to the Abortion Law Reform Association and wanted a test case to confront the courts—came to St. Mary's and warned him not to perform the procedure. Bourne told the police he took great umbrage at their attempt to dictate how he should best care for his patients, and that, anyway, he already had operated on the girl and they could arrest him if they thought it warranted. The attorney general soon brought forward a highly publicized case against Bourne, which carried the threat of a life sentence. The jury acquitted the esteemed obstetrician, and the legal decision for the next four decades gave protection to U.K. doctors willing to perform abortions if they believed that a pregnancy put either a woman's physical or mental health in danger.

I recount this story because it once again demonstrates the odd overlap between miscarriage and abortion: Today, St. Mary's Hospital serves as the world's largest recurrent miscarriage clinic, seeing as many as one thousand new patients annually. Lesley Regan keeps her office and laboratory in the Mint Wing, a cluster of dirty brown brick buildings adjacent to Paddington Station. Originally built as stables, the structure still has the ramps that once took horses to the second floor.

Regan moves at a steady clip, and though she is unfailingly polite to the people who incessantly ask for her time, she has a sharp tongue. Yet she also has a compassionate, sincere demeanor, and she generously pours her heart into her work. She keeps several quotations on her office walls that offer telling glimpses into her personality. One reads, "I'm 51 percent Sweetheart and 49 percent Bitch. Don't Push It." Another slightly modifies a famous admonition from John F. Kennedy: "I forgive my enemies but remember their names." And she displays this Samuel Beckett advice, particularly apropos for both recurrent miscarriage clinicians and patients: "No matter. Try again. Fail again. Fail better."

In the early 1980s, Regan worked at a hospital affiliated with the University of Cambridge and met many patients who had had miscarriages. "They all asked the same question," Regan told me. "Why did it happen?" She quickly noted that the stock replies of "It's nature's way" and "It's a chromosomal abnormality" did little to comfort most people. "No matter the intelligence of the couple; that wasn't a satisfying answer," she said. So Regan studied the potential immune causes of miscarriage—each of which she ultimately dismissed—and in the early 1990s began to specialize in recurrent miscarriage. By the end of the decade she had become a world authority on the topic, publishing a steady stream of well-regarded, rigorously designed clinical studies. She also wrote my favorite miscarriage book for the lay reader, *Miscarriage: What Every Woman Needs to Know, A Positive New Approach*, and allowed Britain's Channel 4 to spend nine months in the clinic shooting an unparalleled, two-hour documentary, *Staying Alive: Tales of Miscarriage*.

Unlike Mary Stephenson and Danny Schust, Regan works with a team of miscarriage specialists, which explains how they handle such a huge caseload. In July 2003, I spent a week observing Regan and her colleagues at work, which included watching them run a clinic for women who have had more than three miscarriages, an early pregnancy clinic for patients during their first trimester, and a prenatal clinic at which they follow their "graduates" from the second trimester all the way to term. Several of the doctors also work in the laboratory, and all of them help write the reams of scientific papers that the team churns out, including one 1997 publication that backed the tender-loving-care thesis: Of 160 pregnant women who received supportive care in the first trimester, 74 percent carried to term versus 49 percent of 41 women who did not receive special care.

An international team of physicians runs the Recurrent Miscarriage Clinic and the Early Pregnancy Clinic: Safaa El Gaddal grew up in Sudan, May Backos in Iraq, Raj Rai in Guyana, and Jan Brosens in Belgium. Their patient base is equally diverse. Pamphlets on the wall of the waiting room explain various tests and procedures in Cantonese, Bengali, Punjabi, Urdu, Gujarati, and other languages. One morning, as I sat and observed the first batch of patients who arrived, I noticed a sari-wrapped Indian woman with a red bindi dot on her forehead flanked by an African woman with a brightly colored head wrap and a big, blond Brit with a husband who looked like a hooligan.

A clock hangs on the wall of each examination room that the clinicians use to meet with the patients. Each of the battery-operated clocks had the wrong time when I visited, and no two were the same. In the world of recurrent miscarriage, clocks matter tremendously, but not the clocks that track the passing of minutes and hours and set themselves to the Royal Observatory in Greenwich. Rather, the biological clock dominates, with ovulatory cycles and the inexorable depletion of eggs determining the meaning of time.

Before opening her exam room door for the first patient of the day, Regan told me that she, too, had put off having children, not becoming pregnant until thirty-seven. "I started very late," she said. And Regan, forty-seven, recounted a serious run-in she had with the miscarriage demons.

Six weeks into her pregnancy, Regan attended a meeting with two dozen colleagues at the Royal Society of Medicine. "I was suddenly aware that something was coming down my leg," said Regan. "It was just one of those horrible situations. I thought I must be miscarrying. Half of me wanted to get help, and the other didn't want anyone to know about it." Regan, afraid to stand, discreetly managed to speak to the only other woman there, who helped find towels so that she could wrap herself and drive home. "I was convinced I'd lost the pregnancy," said Regan.

She phoned her obstetrician, who asked her to come in the next day, a Saturday. "I thought it was a waste, but I went," she said. As it turned out, Regan carried twin girls to term, and she suspects that the blood might have been from her losing a triplet (multiples frequently "vanish" early in pregnancy). "I'm very sympathetic to people who are bleeding," Regan told me. "They can't control what's happening, and they can't control their emotions."

A couple entered the room, and Regan made the introductions. "This lady is forty-one years young," Regan said. The woman had intermittent high levels of follicle-stimulating hormone, and that, coupled with her irregular cycles, indicated that her eggs were running low. She had had six miscarriages and tried everything from Clomid to in vitro fertilization. Regan suggested she try Clomid again, cautioning that it can lead to multiples. "That's not the issue at all," the woman said. "It's the miscarriages."

Regan gently tried to explain the situation more bluntly. "I don't think at this particular moment you're likely to have a pregnancy because you're not ovulating, and unless we get your hormones more fine-tuned, I don't think we're going to get any embryos to implant," she said.

They went back and forth about all the tests the woman has done, and Regan kept pressing her to make a decision about how she wanted to proceed. Finally, a hint exasperated, Regan cut to the chase. "I don't think you have an awful lot of time," she said. "I don't want to have this conversation in December when your FSH level is consistently high, and you say, 'Why didn't you tell me?' A lot of this is guesswork because you're not inside those ovaries and you can't see what the eggs are like. If I had a test that could tell me whether this next pregnancy was going to work or not, I'd be on my way to a Nobel Prize or a fortune." Regan stressed that she did not want to push the woman into taking Clomid, and ended the consultation by suggesting that she give it more thought.

When the couple left the room, Regan shook her head. "I'm very supportive, but they're a bit unkind on their partners," she said. "The bloke knows exactly what's going on. This is the third or fourth conversation I've had with her like this."

Next came a thirty-five-year-old woman who first visited the clinic one year earlier after having three miscarriages. A thorough workup detected high levels of antiphospholipid antibodies, and the woman had tried heparin and aspirin for the past ten months, but had yet to conceive. "My gut is to try IVF or increase my egg production," said the woman, who had her hair in pigtails and looked younger than her age. British health regulations allow women to see IVF specialists only after three years of infertility, Regan explained, noting that a private practice would charge £3,000 (about $5,500).

"I've got three thousand pounds," the woman said.

"My advice would be to do nothing for three or four months," said Regan. "You have a diagnosis of why your miscarriages occurred. I don't think there's anything to suggest you have to do IVF."

They discussed antiphospholipid antibodies in more detail, and then Regan asked whether they had a plan.

"Yeah, come back in December," she said.

"Are you happy about that?"

"I would have liked it to be sooner," she replied.

"I think you're doing yourself a disservice," said Regan.

TLC comes in different flavors, including tough tender-loving care.

I switched to watch Raj Rai, who serves his TLC in the unhurried manner of a therapist who creates the illusion that, for the brief session he has allotted you, you and he have all the time in the world. Rai sat alone, studying the chart of a thirty-three-year-old who had a happier circumstance than the ones Regan took on that morning—yet the case still had its complexities. The woman, who had been diagnosed as having antiphospholipid syndrome after she had three miscarriages, now was six weeks pregnant. Rai normally would have prescribed aspirin and heparin, but she had epilepsy and a brain aneurysm, a ballooning of an artery that occurs because of a weakening of the blood vessel wall. "No one will commit themselves to saying heparin is safe," Rai told me, noting that its blood-thinning properties could cause serious harm to her.

The woman entered, her partner in tow, and immediately pulled from her handbag a bottle of aspirin.

"Who started you on that?" asked Rai.

"I did," she said.

She then pulled out a bottle of folic acid as well as pregnancy vitamins. Rai smiled, and nodded.

He explained that their research had shown that pregnant women with antiphospholipid syndrome who took aspirin alone had a 40 percent success rate, four times that of those who had the condition and took nothing. Adding heparin boosts the success rate to 70 percent, he said. "But you have to balance the risks against the rewards," he said. "In your case the risk is ruptured vessels."

The news did not faze the woman, who explained that she had had an angiogram last year, and the aneurysm had resolved itself.

I could see the worry disappear from Rai's face. "Oh, that makes life a lot easier," he said. "I think we should start heparin. We can start that today." Heparin, he explained, appears to help with implantation. Just to be safe, given her history, he suggested stopping it at twenty-four weeks, by which time the implantation process has finished.

The woman heaved a sigh.

"Does that make sense?" asked Rai.

"Yes, I'm just nervous," she said.

"The important thing is to make a plan, but plans can change," said Rai.

"Is there anything I shouldn't do, like moving around too much?" she asked.

"You should not have bed rest," said Rai. "It's a way to build false hopes."

"Some people say don't be too positive," she replied.

"The most important thing is to support each other," Rai said.

"We went through a lot last year," she said, starting to cry.

Her partner rubbed her knee. "It makes us stronger, doesn't it?" he said.

"It's a bit of a shock," she said, wiping away tears. "I'm supposed to be up here because I wasn't getting pregnant."

"I'm sure we'll get there in the end," said Rai.

"I used to have dreams of miscarriage. Each time," the woman said. "This time, I haven't."

Rai smiled at her as she sobbed.

"I *am* happy," she said. "I'm sorry."

"What are you going to do the rest of the day?" Rai asked.

"Panic."

The last patient I observed with Rai, a thirty-eight-year-old woman who had had seventeen miscarriages and one ectopic pregnancy, came in with her husband. He had the looks of a longshoreman but the gentle way of someone who knew every avenue of miscarriage hell.

"If you want our life story, you're going to need more ink," he told me as I began to scribble notes.

Rai reviewed the woman's charts and then suggested that she might want to have a hysteroscopy to look for scar tissue that they could then remove.

"We're looking at surrogacy," the woman said.

"Unless you can see different in your heart of hearts," said her husband.

Rai explained that the quality of her eggs likely was declining with her age, and that she might have better luck with an egg donated from another woman.

"That won't actually be my baby," the woman said.

"Not genetically," said Rai.

"That's not an option for me," she said sternly.

"Explore all the options," said Rai. "But if you're using your eggs, that might be where the problem lies." He then explained to them a relatively new experimental technique, preimplantation genetic diagnosis, which, was used in in vitro fertilization. He cautioned that it probably would not help them. Doctors remove one cell from the embryo when it is at about the eight-cell stage and check the chromosomes. They then transfer only chromosomally normal embryos into the mother. Rai explained that if she had a problem with, say, her uterine lining, preimplantation genetic diagnosis would not help. He suggested they consider adoption, too.

"What you're saying is there's no way she's going to do it with her egg," her husband cut in.

Rai slowly explained that several factors caused miscarriage, and said, given her history and her age . . .

"Why was I getting to twelve to fourteen weeks and then losing it?" she interrupted, her voice catching.

"That's life, isn't it?" her husband said.

Rai asked them if they knew about implantation, and in unison they said "no," so he gave them an extended biology lesson, complete with drawings. "In your case, we're not sure of anything," Rai said.

He then urged them to think hard about their options, including a donor egg. "Who's the parent?" Rai asked. "The people whose genetic information it is? Or is it the people who take care of the child? You can't discuss this in twenty minutes."

"We've had nineteen years discussing this," said the woman.

They talked about surrogacy, which Rai said was "a bit of a minefield."

"You can do no more, can you?" asked the husband.

"That's exactly right," said Rai.

"If you were in our shoes, what would you do?"

"I'm not a big fan of surrogacy," Rai said. "Reproductive medicine is a business—"

"What you're saying is they're thieves," the husband interrupted.

Rai said nothing, and the husband filled the silence with a short aside about his wife's miscarriage history. "One night we were watching the telly," he said. "That was the first time she miscarried. I said, 'Let's just wait until the show is over.' How stupid can you be?"

As they thanked Rai and said their good-byes, the wet-eyed woman said, "I'm very disappointed."

Anxiety again filled the air when I visited the Early Pregnancy Clinic the next day, but the concerns predictably had switched from the worry about becoming pregnant to the worry of being pregnant. I sat with Safaa El Gaddal as she met with patient after patient who wanted help decoding the risks that their baby would have a survivable chromosomal abnormality such as Down syndrome. El Gaddal, a fan of Stephen King novels who has a big, easy laugh, spoke to each patient in a jargonless conversation that effortlessly seemed to translate bizarre-sounding concepts like risk ratios into plain English.

During the first trimester, blood tests can screen for proteins and hormones that indicate the likelihood of a chromosomal abnormality and other aberrations. These markers, combined with ultrasound measurements of the nape of the neck called the nuchal fold, can predict nearly 90 percent of Down syndrome cases. Because abnormalities increase with the mother's age, clinics now routinely factor that in when helping a couple assess their risks. None of these indicators have the nearly 100 percent predictive power of either chorionic villi sampling or amniocentesis, yet they also do not pose the risk of miscarriage presented by those invasive procedures. Although that miscarriage risk runs to only 1 percent or less, many women who have had repeated losses, Shannon included, understandably decline the option to test the fetus directly, leaving them much more reliant upon the markers. "When they come up with nothing, it's reassuring, but when it's in the middle, it's disorienting," El Gaddal told a thirty-eight-year-old woman whose workup suggested that her baby had a 1 in 247 risk of having a problem.

A thirty-nine-year-old woman then came in and explained that her two-year-old son had accidentally sliced her eye with his fingernail while trying to hug her. "When you have children, you should have crash helmets," she quipped. But she had serious qualms about an antibiotic eye drop a doctor had prescribed and wanted El Gaddal's assurance that it would not hurt her twelve-week-old fetus.

"I wouldn't worry about your baby," said El Gaddal, stressing that she would not recommend the eye drops later in the pregnancy.

"That's brilliant," said the woman.

Seven years earlier, a cyst led to the removal of a fallopian tube. She then had three miscarriages in the same year, which led her and her husband to quit trying to have children. "We were just going to go get dogs and do a bed and breakfast in the middle of Scotland," she said. Her general practitioner then referred her to the St. Mary's Recurrent Miscarriage Clinic, and she decided to have another go at it after the doctors diagnosed her as having antiphospholipid syndrome. "Last time I was here often," she said to me. "I was part of the staff." She credits the care with her son's birth. "We wouldn't have had him otherwise," she said matter-of-factly.

"So do you have a dog now?" El Gaddal asked.

"Gosh, now that's out the window," she said, and both laughed.

I joined May Backos for the rest of the afternoon.

I had asked Backos a few days earlier what it felt like, from the doctor's perspective, to work in a clinic devoted to women who have repeatedly miscarried. "Can you imagine seeing ten patients who are completely distraught and trying to get them to term and convincing them there's hope?" she asked me. "They've all seen all this trauma. It's very stressful for us. We need a day to calm down. But at the end of the day, when you see someone rejoice at having a baby, it's very rewarding."

Often at the Early Pregnancy Clinic, Backos has to inform a patient that she has miscarried yet again, but not today. "Thank goodness," she told me.

Backos has a calm, wise demeanor, and I saw it seriously tested by an obviously well educated patient and her partner who both had strong misgivings about Western medicine—and the people who provide it.

"You're pregnant now," said Backos good-naturedly to her last patients of the day. "Congratulations."

"I'm forty-four," the woman replied. "Congratulations may be a bit wrong."

"There's a heartbeat," said Backos brightly. "That's good."

The woman, who also had antiphospholipid syndrome, explained that she had no interest in taking heparin. She had altered her diet after learning of her diagnosis, eating mainly raw vegetables and fruit, fish for protein, garlic to thin her blood, and several vitamin supplements. "When we decided after long consultations here that we didn't want to try heparin, we stopped trying to have a baby," she continued. "This pregnancy is unplanned. We are in a bit of a dilemma about what to do." The woman explained that someone she knew had done the heparin treatment and had a small baby that was not growing properly. She also worried about what heparin would do to her. "I'm really anxious," she said. What if she had a car wreck and then had to wait for the heparin to clear her body before surgeons could operate on her? Wouldn't heparin mean she would have to have a C-section, ruling out the prospects of her having a "proper birth"?

Backos remained silent.

"There are a lot of anxieties," said the woman, who had become obviously agitated.

"Do you want to talk about it?" Backos finally asked.

She explained that the size of the heparin molecule prevented it from passing to the baby, dismissed the idea that heparin precluded a proper birth, and emphasized that women with *untreated* antiphospholipid syndrome actually had a higher risk of underweight babies. As for the heparin causing dangerous thinning of the blood, Backos said they had seen no such effect in the seven hundred women they had given the drug. "I appreciate the dilemma and what you're going through," Backos said, "but your chromosomal risk actually is bigger than your risk from the antiphospholipid antibodies."

Backos explained that she might consider just taking aspirin, which their studies have shown can lower the risk of miscarrying in women with antiphospholipid syndrome from 90 percent to 60 percent.

"I have a real aversion to taking medicine," the woman replied.

"If this pregnancy were to work, we'd be happy, wouldn't we?" asked Backos.

"Of course," said the man.

The woman agreed. "If we decide not to do heparin, will the hospital support me?" she asked.

"Of course we'd support you," said Backos. "All the way through. We don't push heparin. If you want to think about it more, maybe just start aspirin."

The woman began to cry.

"I haven't had a drug inside of me for twenty years," she said.

Backos suggested that she have a blood sample tested with the thromboelastograph, which measures clotting strength. Antiphospholipid antibodies, she explained, might not be her only problem. The idea remained experimental, but new evidence from a prospective study the clinic did in women who did *not* have antiphospholipid syndrome strongly suggested that if blood forms clots too readily—possibly because of an excess of thrombin, an enzyme critical in the clotting process—it can lead to implantation problems. A new study the clinic had under way would attempt to evaluate whether treating with a double dose of daily baby aspirin would reduce the clotting strength and decrease the miscarriage rate. Backos asked whether she wanted them to do her "blood clotting."

"Will you tell me the results?" the woman asked.

"If it's high, would you take aspirin?" replied Backos.

"What about the safety of aspirin?" asked her partner.

The meeting ended cordially, even warmly, with no clear resolution.

May Backos was tired. She had seen eight patients today, and had worked the Recurrent Miscarriage Clinic the day before. We talked about this and that, and then she said, "I believe it's the support you get here more than anything else." She was not referring to her last patient of the day. But then again, maybe, without meaning to, she was.

11

······---------······

MIRACLE BABIES

IN 1932, THE MEXICAN ARTIST FRIDA KAHLO PAINTED A gruesome self-portrait of a miscarriage. She lies naked on a bed labeled "Henry Ford Hospital, Detroit," where the miscarriage took place. A pool of blood stains the white sheets of the neatly made bed. A large tear falls from her left eye. A perfectly formed baby boy floats above Kahlo like a balloon, tethered to a red rope that she holds in one hand. Another red rope in her hand has a snail tied to its end, a symbol that this miscarriage, one of at least two she suffered, had occurred at an excruciatingly slow pace.

Henry Ford Hospital, also known as The Flying Bed, is the world's most famous artistic depiction of miscarriage. The image captures the tragedy of losing a baby in the making, and it leaves viewers with a deep compassion for Kahlo and, for women in particular, a sense of anxiety for themselves. I found the image on several Web sites, and printed a copy of it that I kept on my desk for months as I researched and wrote this book. The complexity of the painting intrigued me, but, more than that, it seared something deep inside, constantly reminding me of the raw pain, the confusion at the injustice, the rage at the helplessness that miscarriage made me feel.

But during the past few years, I have witnessed equally disturbing images that made me appreciate how a miscarriage, even an emotionally devastating one, can be a merciful, fortunate event. And one early-morning visit to the main hospital run by the University of California at San Diego stands out.

At the invitation of Kurt Benirschke, the esteemed reproductive pathologist whose pioneering work helped establish the link between chromosomal abnormalities and miscarriage, I entered the section of the hospital cafeteria reserved for doctors. Once every other week, Benirschke and his colleagues hold a prenatal diagnosis meeting, a briskly paced review of problematic pregnancies they have recently encountered. The meeting opened with Benirschke showing photographs he had taken during an autopsy of a twenty-three-week-old baby. "It's a mangled fetus, as usual," he said, introducing the case. They next discussed a fetus with trisomy that was missing a leg, and then a fourteen-year-old mother who lost one of two twins at sixteen weeks who had no legs at all growing from its pelvis. Then came a dwarfed fetus with a lethal condition called short rib polydactyly syndrome and twins in which one had Down syndrome.

"OK, buckle up," said Benirschke.

He described a twenty-eight-year-old mother, who had four children and "multiple" miscarriages, who had terminated a pregnancy at twenty-two weeks because the baby had a malformed skull. "There are no bones in there whatsoever," said Benirschke, showing a photo he had taken. At the autopsy, he also found an IUD, the intrauterine device meant to prevent pregnancy, in the placenta. "It didn't work," he said, shaking his head. The doctors decided she might have an abnormality known as gonadal mosaicism, in which some of her eggs carry abnormal complements of chromosomes before meiosis occurs.

Subsequent cases they viewed and discussed over coffee and doughnuts included a triploidy, thirteen-week-old conjoined twins who had just two hands growing from one trunk, a suspected trisomy 18, an overgrown umbilical cord that was almost as large as the fetus, and a baby without a bladder. By the end of the meeting, I had concluded that most every case I saw represented the failure of the miscarriage mechanism, which, had it functioned properly, would have detected these problems early in the first trimester, sparing the child and the parents tremendous suffering. The cumulative impact of these images also reinforced my conviction that every child who comes to term without any significant health problems represents a miracle.

While researching this book, I spoke with nearly one hundred people about their miscarriages, and many a woman who subsequently carried to term, Shannon included, referred to her child as a "miracle baby." I do see something miraculous about babies born to women who have suffered several losses. Given that a miracle, by definition, transcends the laws of nature, this usage may seem absurd: miscarriage much of the time is nature's way, the superb gatekeeper that humans have evolved to discard all but the most fit embryos and fetuses, undoubtedly improving life for individuals and for the species at large. Yet miscarriage also can purposelessly end many a life prematurely. And for people who experience several losses—typically with no knowledge of why they happened—miscarriage can seem particularly cruel, with each one inevitably pushing the dream of carrying to term further and further away, leaving couples with implacable hungers and psyches as scarred as Frida Kahlo's. When miscarriage veterans who do keep trying and manage, whether by chance, medical intervention, or adoption, to fill the crib they had stored in the rafters, I can well understand why they feel particularly blessed. I am, after all, one of them.

In my journeys through the world of miscarriage, I came across a few cases, that, more than any of the others, defied the odds. Although they might suggest, anecdotally, interventions that work or that pointedly do not, I think each one offers an abundance of another force that, like love, science cannot accurately gauge: hope. Here then are four unrelated stories that twisted my head and my soul, expanding my notion of the possible.

In 1999, a thirty-six-year-old woman in Melbourne, Australia, decided to try in vitro fertilization after seven years of failed attempts to become pregnant. The woman had a history of infertility, not miscarriage, but her experience has important implications for the future treatment of recurrent losses, as it offers a new strategy that aims to eliminate chromosomally abnormal embryos from the equation.

After doctors fertilized her eggs with her husband's sperm, the couple ended up with eight embryos. During four separate procedures, doctors at her infertility clinic, Melbourne IVF, transferred embryos made from this same batch of eggs into her uterus. None implanted.

The woman opted to try again, but this time the clinic checked the chromosomes in each of the nine embryos they made, using the procedure known as preimplantation genetic diagnosis. Devised in the early 1990s to determine whether an embryo inherited genes that cause diseases like cystic fibrosis or Huntington's, preimplantation genetic diagnosis, or PGD, has become commonplace at clinics worldwide—and a lightning rod for ethicists who worry about designer babies and the like. Many fertility clinics now offer PGD, too; in vitro fertilization frequently fails because the embryo had an unusual number of chromosomes.

To assess the chromosomes of the Melbourne woman, scientists, led by the geneticist Leeanda Wilton, removed one cell from each three-day-old embryo. They then turned to probes that could seek out specific chromosomes and label them with fluorescent tags. This fishing expedition—which appropriately goes by the acronym FISH (fluorescence in situ hybridization)—had a critical limitation: for technical reasons, they could check only five of the twenty-three pairs of chromosomes in each cell. They chose the ones that most frequently caused trisomies in miscarriages.

Melbourne IVF transferred the only two of the nine embryos that tested chromosomally normal. Neither took.

The woman went through yet a third cycle. This time, Wilton took no chances and turned to comparative genomic hybridization, the technique adopted from cancer research which Mary Stephenson and her Vancouver miscarriage clinic recently had begun using to karyotype miscarriages. Comparative genomic hybridization, unlike FISH, can detect the presence of all twenty-three pairs of chromosomes in an embryo. This technique does have its own technical shortcoming: it requires five days to complete, which means clinics must freeze and then thaw the embryos, which studies have shown destroys at least 30 percent of them. Still, comparative genomic hybridization can supply more information than FISH. "It just makes sense," Wilton told me. "It's obvious."

Wilton and her team harvested fourteen eggs, eleven of which they successfully inseminated. They transferred two embryos that FISH deemed normal, but the woman did not become pregnant. For five of the embryos, they turned to comparative genomic hybridization. Only one had a normal karyotype. (Interestingly, one of the abnormal ones would have passed the FISH test.)

Wilton had little hope that the one normal embryo they found with comparative genomic hybridization would work. "It wasn't a particularly great-looking embryo," she said. "It is not the one that would have been transferred by embryologists." Still, they transferred this single embryo, and, for the first time, the patient had a clinically viable pregnancy. As Wilton and her colleagues reported in the *New England Journal of Medicine* in 2001, their patient gave birth to a healthy daughter.

Preimplantation genetic diagnosis, let alone comparative genomic hybridization, has yet to prove its worth in a carefully designed study with patients who have miscarriage problems, and Mary Stephenson, for one, doubts it will. She pointed to a study in her clinic of 285 patients: women under thirty-six years of age who had recurrent miscarriage had more chromosomally *normal* losses than a control group of women who had no history of repeated losses; this sample indicates that younger women who have repeated losses, as a group, more frequently have underlying problems unrelated to abnormal chromosomes. Providing these women with chromosomally normal embryos might have no impact on their ability to carry to term.

As for women thirty-six or older, Stephenson and colleagues found that this group had the same amount of chromosomally abnormal miscarriages as the controls, suggesting that the aging process, rather than some unique aberration, accounted for their losses. This older group, which has Mother Time staring them down, logically might opt for preimplantation genetic diagnosis to increase their odds of transferring a chromosomally normal embryo, but Stephenson questioned this logic, too, for reasons of cost—IVF itself can generate thousands of dollars of medical bills—practicality, and safety.

Preimplantation genetic diagnosis removes one of the six to ten cells typically found in a three-day-old embryo. Several studies have shown that an IVF embryo can have different chromosomes in different cells. This so-called mosaicism means that a cell, even one tested with comparative genomic hybridization, could have normal chromosomes, but the embryo might contain other, chromosomally abnormal cells that would come to dominate as it grew, leading to a miscarriage or even an abnormal child.

In 2000, two sobering studies, one from Wilton's group and the other from Dagan Wells and Joy Delhanty of the University of London Medical School, reported that chromosomally normal IVF embryos remained the exception rather than the rule. Each study had twelve "surplus" embryos, donated by patients, that had between three and eight cells. The two groups both used comparative genomic hybridization to analyze as many cells from each embryo as possible. Combined, they analyzed 129 cells from the twenty-four embryos. Nearly two-thirds of the embryos proved mosaic. Only six embryos had completely normal chromosomes. Equally startling, many of the abnormal ones appeared normal to the trained eye, the most common method of selecting embryos for a transfer. Evidence exists that the ovarian stimulation and the test-tube culturing used in assisted reproduction of an embryo can trigger mosaicism.

On the safety side of the equation, health problems have not surfaced in studies of children born after preimplantation genetic diagnosis. But Stephenson noted that removing a cell from an embryo crosses into a new frontier. (As of June 2000, only about four hundred pregnancies had occurred worldwide after preimplantation genetic diagnosis.) "Can we really say it's doing no harm?" she asked me. "We don't really know."

Even taking all these red flags into consideration, I remain flabbergasted at what preimplantation genetic diagnosis did for this Melbourne woman. No one knows whether the luck of the draw might have worked in her favor without screening the embryos, but the odds were wildly stacked against her. Preimplantation genetic diagnosis found only four normal embryos out of twenty tested. Comparative genomic hybridization further uncovered one aneuploid embryo that would have tested normal with FISH. Add to this quantitative argument for screening embryos the qualitative one: by the time doctors transferred the one embryo that ended up coming to term, the patient had endured three cycles of ovarian stimulation and egg retrieval, and six transfers of twelve embryos, which then failed.

At this state of the art, I share Stephenson's hold-your-horses perspective about the enthusiasm now sweeping through IVF clinics about preimplantation genetic diagnosis, and comparative genomic hybridization in particular. But I see the promise, too. Roughly seven out of ten transferred embryos miscarry, with an even higher failure rate for older women, who typically have more chromosomally abnormal eggs. The birth of this Australian girl suggests that as scientists improve their ability to select healthy embryos, in vitro fertilization will move from a crap shoot to a predictable procedure. Preimplantation genetic diagnosis, theoretically, also should allow higher success rates with fewer embryos transferred, reducing the risk of in vitro fertilization leading to twins or higher multiples.

Leeanda Wilton predicted other, less readily apparent benefits from preimplantation genetic diagnosis. Given better tools to distinguish the chromosomally normal from the abnormal, scientists will gain a better understanding of what a healthy embryo looks like, possibly eclipsing the need for any invasive analysis. "What I'd actually hope in the long term is that we wouldn't do nearly as much preimplantation genetic diagnosis as we now do," she told me. Wilton also pointed out that more precise genetic information will allow people to assess their reproductive fate more accurately. "I think it's going to make us practice better medicine in terms of helping patients make decisions more quickly based on better information," she said, telling me the story of a patient whose nineteen analyzed embryos—to a one—were chromosomally abnormal. The patient finally relied on a donor egg, became pregnant right off the bat, and carried to term.

Reproductive medicine moves at a breakneck pace, routinely racing experimental procedures into standard practice long before scientific evidence alone would warrant. Preimplantation genetic diagnosis for aneuploidy may well have become the latest example of this phenomenon, and people shopping for reproductive help would do themselves a favor if they kept that in mind. Yet it also makes sense to keep a close eye on these screening technologies. If they pass muster, wannabe parents will have a new place to turn.

· · ·

Many couples I met at recurrent miscarriage clinics had dramatic, traumatic, tragic tales to tell that nevertheless had happy endings. But the harrowing travail I heard from Shelley Adams, who had serious health complications of her own—as well as a wonderful ability to articulate the odd nuances of miscarriage—left me with a renewed sense of the word *miracle*.

Shelley and her husband, Destry, got pregnant the first month they tried. Recently married, Adams, then thirty, remembers that she tested positive on a home pregnancy test on Labor Day 1995. "I had morning sickness, tender breasts. Everything seemed to be OK," Adams said. A buyer for a school district in a Vancouver suburb, Adams told her co-workers and her family. "Everyone was very excited." But within four days, cramps arrived, and at eight weeks she spotted. An ultrasound at thirteen weeks captured no fetus. "It's the mundaneness of how it happens that's so boggling," said Adams, who had gone to the clinic with her father because Destry had to work that day. "Who ever suspects that's going to happen?"

Her father drove her home and suggested that he stay until Destry returned. "My dad was really great, but he didn't know what to say or what to do," remembered Adams. "I said I wanted to be alone." Destry had left work, stopping on the way home to buy her flowers.

Not long after her father left, Adams hemorrhaged. She phoned 911.

"I'm bleeding," she said, moments before she passed out. She awoke in an ambulance.

A few months later, in early 1996, she became pregnant for the second time and soon started spotting. The embryo had died at seven weeks. Adams checked into the hospital for a dilation and curettage after dinnertime, and the day nurse said she could spend the night. A new night nurse had a different idea, and at 3 A.M., woke Adams and told her to find a ride home or they would charge her $1,500 for the stay.

"I can't believe at three A.M. you're telling me I've got to leave the hospital," Adams protested. "Who the hell is coming in here?" But she left, livid.

An emotional state "beyond depression" leveled Adams. "I'm the roller coaster queen—I could live on a roller coaster," she told me. But miscarriage exacted a sharp price. "It's so not how you thought your life was going to be. It just doesn't happen to people like me." It also stunned this wry, forthcoming woman to find how her sad news tongue-tied many people. "It was a silence because they don't want to upset you," she said. "It seemed kind of cold. 'I'm sorry' would have at least acknowledged that this was a life that just wasn't going to happen."

Right away, Shelley and Destry tried and, come April, the same story replayed itself: pregnant, spotting at seven weeks, miscarriage. Adams knew about the recurrent miscarriage clinic run by Stephenson at Children and Women's Health Centre, and felt relieved that she finally had the required three losses to receive a referral.

Adams first came to the clinic in the fall of 1996. "It was finally a place where people totally understood," she said. "I had *What to Expect When You're Expecting*. Not once did that book have anything to do with me." Like many of the patients I met at the Vancouver clinic, she developed a deep bond with her doctor. "We all love Mary," she said.

The standard battery of blood tests revealed moderately elevated antiphospholipid antibodies. Stephenson put Adams on heparin and baby aspirin. She became pregnant for the fourth time the next spring, and when she came to the clinic for her first visit, they found a heartbeat, the first she had ever seen. At her eight-week visit, the heartbeat had vanished. "It was crushing," she said, particularly because they finally had arrived at a diagnosis that purported to explain the other losses. "But at least I knew right away, and Mary was there, and there was emotional support with Edwina," Stephenson's head nurse. Her father had taken her to the clinic, and he charmed her with his response to the news. "Let's go have a cigarette and a coffee," he said.

Karyotypes from two of her miscarriages had shown that both embryos, one female, one male, had normal chromosomes.

Miscarriage can create a whirlwind of funk, and, with each successive one, the twister can start up again and twirl faster still. "I felt helpless to stop it," said Adams. "And the more losses you have, the more people look at you like, Ohmigod, why are you doing this? Are you stupid? Why are you inflicting this pain?" And the serene, contented image on the faces of the pregnant women smiling in the magazines: forget it. "The sad thing is, you can never enjoy the joy of it," said Adams. "I never had the joy of shopping for maternity clothes. I never got to stand and hold my belly and have that picture."

Instead of bailing, Adams did the opposite. "After that loss, I said I'm going to do whatever I can to have a baby," she said. "I didn't want to look back in ten years and say, Why didn't I try that drug? If I wasn't going to have a child, it was because I had exhausted every avenue." Yet at the same time she vowed to herself that once she had explored it to the hilt, she would quit. "I wasn't going to be the kind of woman who just keeps doing it, having fifty-five miscarriages."

Out of altruism more than anything else, Adams joined a Stephenson study with a different kind of heparin. Its lower molecular weight required fewer doses and potentially had fewer side effects. In the fall of 1998, she became pregnant but soon miscarried. "Same old, same old," she told me. Except this time, her internal whirlwind did not blow. "By this point, you're steeled to it, emotionally shut down so you don't go crazy," she said. "Men get lost in the whole process."

The respite did not last. A boss blanched at her request for a few days off because he said she already had had too many. "You know what? I was in a frickin' hospital, having a D and C," she said to me, still clearly exasperated. She took a leave of absence, and then quit to work in her father's business. "I was hypersensitive to anything," she said.

Her sixth pregnancy came in the summer of 1999, but at a work seminar with her father she began to hemorrhage, which led her back to the hospital for another D and C. A karyotype announced a chromosomally normal girl. In one three-day stretch, Adams read the entire Bible. "All I saw was 'barren womb, barren womb, barren womb.'"

Stephenson suggested what amounted to a last-ditch effort: add intravenous immunoglobulin to the aspirin and heparin. Once every four weeks, Adams spent eight hours at the clinic, receiving infusions of these pooled antibodies, which some evidence suggests might help people who have antiphospholipid antibodies and yet still miscarry while taking heparin and aspirin. She started taking progesterone, too. "My understanding was that it couldn't hurt," said Adams. On New Year's of the millennium, Shelley Adams became pregnant for the seventh time in less than five years.

Six weeks into the pregnancy, Adams started to hemorrhage yet again. "It feels like your guts are going to be spewed out." An ultrasound revealed a heartbeat, but a blood clot had formed in her uterus. "I've seen only one bigger," Stephenson told her.

"We all decided the worst," said Adams, who went straight from the ultrasound to the antepartum ward, which cares for high-risk pregnant women before they go into labor. Adams stayed for one week. "Being there was really comforting in a really scary way," she said. "I didn't have to move and feed myself." When she returned home, horribly ill with morning sickness, she put herself on bed rest for another four weeks.

By twelve weeks, Adams had become more confident, as weekly ultrasounds showed that the baby had continued to grow, and the blood clot had started to shrink. The next week, she passed a large clot. "That was not good, but I went for an ultrasound, and everything was OK, which was almost as shocking as it's not," she said.

Lying in bed at eighteen weeks, Adams felt a trickle between her legs and was certain she had started to bleed, but it did not look like blood. Worried that her water had prematurely broken, she and Destry hurried to the hospital, where doctors swabbed and tested the liquid for the pH of amniotic fluid. The test came back negative. Go home, it's nothing, they told her. "I was reassured, but in the back of my mind, I thought, Nah," she said. Fluid continued to leak and she returned to the hospital the next day, at which point the amniotic fluid test turned positive.

"I hate to tell you, but you're going to have this baby," the doctor said, explaining that there was nothing they could do and that she should just return home.

This cannot be happening, Adams thought. The couple refused to leave. "I'm not going home to miscarry my eighteen-week-old baby," she told them. "We were very adamant that we weren't leaving, so they finally put me in a room." They gave the baby a 5 percent chance of surviving.

Week after week, ultrasound after ultrasound, the baby's heart kept beating and its bones kept growing. Adams developed gestational diabetes. At twenty-nine weeks she checked herself out. "I could not stand hospital food one more day," she said. Yet a short four days later, she found herself back at the hospital, in labor. Because her membranes had ruptured prematurely, the doctors suspected that she had developed an infection, triggering the early labor. After three days of labor, the doctors performed a cesarean section, and Shelley Adams gave birth to a two-pound, thirteen-ounce girl. "Nobody thought she would live," says Adams. The doctors sent her to the Neonatal Intensive Care Unit, where they put the tiny, bruised baby in what looked like a roasting pan and covered her in plastic wrap.

Shelley and Destry named their daughter Karis, which means "graceful" in Greek.

Karis's lungs, to everyone's surprise, were more developed than they had anticipated. But it remained touch and go. "Every day she was OK was a good day," remembered Adams. The Neonatal Intensive Care Unit would serve as home for the next eight weeks, by which point Karis weighed a hearty five pounds. By the time I met Shelley Adams in July 2003, Karis, a perfectly healthy young girl, was about to celebrate her third birthday. "People say, 'Look what your daughter put you through,'" said Adams, laughing. "My attitude is, Look what I put *her* through."

I spent more than two years interviewing couples about their miscarriages, and, frequently, when describing this project to people at dinner parties and the like, I recount some of the remarkable odysseys I have heard. The story I repeat most frequently is about Claire and Frank, two educated Southern California professionals who asked that I identify them by their middle names.

When Claire was a teenager, her tampons always seemed to leak. "I was a surfer chick who lived at the beach and couldn't understand what was going on," said Claire when we first spoke. "I'd tell my mother and she'd say, Yeah, whatever." A healthy young woman, Claire rarely saw a doctor and waited until she reached college age before she visited a gynecologist, who, she said, "was mystified about what was going on with my anatomy."

Claire's gynecologist discovered that she had a didelphic uterus, the abnormality in which the müllerian ducts fail to fuse, creating two uteri, two cervixes, and, in her case, two distinct vaginal canals separated by muscular tissue called a septum. Until then, Claire had no notion that she had two vaginal openings, as one was much smaller than the other, which explained why a tampon placed in the larger one appeared to leak. At her gynecologist's recommendation, she had the septum that separated the two vaginal canals removed. "I didn't think much of it," she said. "I could use tampons. And because I wasn't sexually active yet, it wasn't an issue."

Claire started to date Frank in 1986, and three years later they moved in together, but they did not marry until 1995, by which time she had turned thirty-four and he was thirty-six. Finally, they started trying to have a family. "I was concerned in the back of my head about this condition," said Claire, who by then had studied her problem and even met other women with uterine anomalies. She also suspected that she had had a miscarriage in a previous relationship: her ovulatory cycle doesn't skip a beat, and she once had an extremely late period.

After several months of failing to conceive, Claire and Frank visited her gynecologist. "I see it all the time," the gynecologist said. "No big deal. One of the uteruses just disappears and you'll have no problem." Around their first wedding anniversary, Claire tested positive on a home pregnancy test, but she miscarried. "It was pretty upsetting, but I'd had friends who'd gone through miscarriages," said Claire. "Frank was more upset. I tried not to deal with the emotional issues. I was sharklike. Just keep moving forward. Keep having a game plan. I always have to have an A, B, and a C option."

Frank, a marathon runner and surfer, has a nice blend of tough and soft, and I found this role reversal thoroughly charming. "Claire was the pillar in this," he told me. "To some extent, the miscarriage process is very binding for the couple, but to some extent it's very lonely. It was very raw on the emotional front for me. And some of those emotions I had to keep to myself because I didn't want to expose her to more than she already was dealing with." Couples share their miscarriages, he said. "It's not a woman's issue. You, me, all the fathers whose hopes were dashed, suffer too."

In December 1996, Claire and Frank made the first of many visits to a fertility specialist. Claire and Frank gave me copies of many of their reproductive medical records, 150 pages of the rich, odd details of fertility, written cryptically in doctor's code, documenting everything from the motility of Frank's sperm to the nuances of Claire's ovulatory cycle—and the size of her right and left cervix. From the outset, their new ob-gyn had serious concerns about Claire's septate uterus, and a scan soon showed that she also had a large fibroid. Blood tests ruled out antiphospholipid syndrome, evidence of infection, or any other abnormality. The doctor recommended surgery, and Claire agreed.

In March 1997, Claire went under the knife, but because she bled more heavily than anticipated when the surgeons resected her septum they could not remove the fibroid. "They nicked her pretty badly," Frank asserted, still angry years later. "I wanted to strangle the doctors. Not only did it lead to bleeding, it created additional scar tissue in the uterus, which we were trying to avoid."

Come late May, Claire suspected another pregnancy and, as a precaution, her doctor prescribed progesterone supplements. A scan a month later showed nothing but an empty sac. "Inevitable abortion," the doctor wrote in shorthand.

At the doctor's request, Claire brought in what her charts refer to as the POC, the products of conception. "I picked a grayish mass out of the toilet," she recalled. "You could see the sac and not much else. I didn't show it to Frank. I felt this need to protect him emotionally." The karyotype, as often happens, yielded no results.

Following her third miscarriage, Claire began taking progesterone, as well as baby aspirin and Clomid. In January 1998, she became pregnant again. In her chart after the first ultrasound scan, the doctor wrote, "Prob. SAb," shorthand for "probably a spontaneous abortion." She miscarried, her fourth, one week later. "I could feel the hormone shifts in my body when I was miscarrying," Claire told me. "I could feel the pregnancy leaving me."

Their fertility specialist recommended that they try lymphocyte immune therapy, and that February Frank started to have regular blood draws so that the doctors could remove his white blood cells and then inject them into Claire. Supposedly, this treatment would stop Claire's immune system from rejecting the babies they made together. "We really did feel the quackery and witchcraft with all this," said Claire. Frank said they were grasping at straws by then. "We had a false sense of anticipation, to be honest." They had no way of knowing that one month after Claire first received an infusion of Frank's white blood cells, a group of experts monitoring the largest, best study ever done of lymphocyte immune therapy quietly stopped the trial because evidence had surfaced that the treatment did not work.

A home pregnancy test turned positive in July 1998. Ten days later, when she went in for her first ultrasound scan, Claire had started to spot, and her doctor suggested bed rest. A week later, the bleeding increased and a stabbing pain emanated from her left side. "Threatened SAb," the doctor wrote in the chart.

That August, Frank's grandmother died, and he flew to her funeral, while Claire stayed home. Claire's pregnancy was the equivalent of a state secret, and he planned to dodge his family's questions about her. "We found that talking about pregnancy with other people and talking about miscarriage made it worse, much, much worse," said Frank. "More people discussing it more often was like pulling scabs off the wound, and it made it bleed more, not heal. As we got older, our family and our friends started putting pressure on us to have kids: 'If nothing's wrong with you, what's the problem?'" quoted Frank. "That pressure is constant and irritating. Patting me on the back: 'Shooting blanks there, buddy?' Fuck you. Who are you? I don't ask what kind of ammunition you have in your gun."

Claire phoned him just as he was leaving with his family for the ceremony. "She was crying and saying, 'I'm miscarrying,'" remembered Frank. "I didn't know what to do."

Claire had a D and C a few weeks later, and a karyotype showed that the embryo had normal chromosomes. "I couldn't understand what nature was doing," said Claire. "There was no explanation for why it happened." The normal karyotype, however, also brought a sense of relief. "Her eggs were good, at least in this case, and if we had good eggs, we could turn them into babies," said Frank. In September, Claire, who by then had had five miscarriages, told her doctor she wanted to try surrogacy. "Burnt out by SAb's," the doctor wrote. "Doesn't want to do HSG [hysterosalpingogram], laparotomy, etc." Claire told me that she also had lost faith in her doctor. "We had lost a lot of time dealing with her because she was so timid." Fortunately, this ob-gyn left the clinic and Claire immediately liked the replacement.

Two weeks later, the couple started the cumbersome process of finding a woman who would carry an embryo made from Claire's egg and Frank's sperm. "We wanted kids so badly," said Claire. "I had done a lot of soul-searching. Is it the pregnancy experience I wanted or children? I wanted children. On the list of A, B, C options, adoption was an F. I grew up with adopted children on my street and saw other issues I didn't want to tackle. I'm also into genealogy. One of my coping skills was to do genealogical research for my family. I ended up joining the Mayflower Society. I found family history all the way back to the abolitionists. It made it all the more important to me to have genetic offspring."

The surrogacy service that Claire and Frank worked with had a drawn-out process that included in-depth interviews with them about their religious faith and what they thought of abortion and reducing multiples. The service then would match them to a woman who had similar beliefs. By the spring of 1999, they had found a surrogate that they both liked, and Claire started injecting hormones to artificially stimulate production of eggs. Doctors harvested ten eggs and made six embryos, transferring two into the surrogate and freezing the other four. The transfer at first seemed to take, based on rising levels of human chorionic gonadotropin, but the hormonal indicator of implantation soon plummeted and the doctors found nothing on an ultrasound scan. The next month, in June 1999, they tried again, transferring the only two of the frozen embryos that survived the thaw. None took. The surrogate, said Frank, "was chomping at the bit and said, 'Let's do it again.'"

Having run out of embryos, the doctors in September 1999 stimulated Claire's ovaries to produce more eggs. Patient "wants to be as aggressive as possible," the doctor noted in Claire's chart. "I felt like a hen with a clutch of eggs," said Claire. "I could barely move." This time, they removed nineteen eggs, transferring four embryos to the surrogate and freezing away another five. The hCG levels steadily climbed, indicating that at least one embryo had implanted.

Claire attended the seven-week ultrasound scan, done in the same room where she had learned of her own miscarriages several times before. The doctor noted that the surrogate had miscarried. The distraught surrogate fainted. "She grew to love us and care about us and she wanted nothing more than to help us have a child," said Claire.

A karyotype of the miscarriage showed that a normal female embryo had implanted. "That was so devastating," said Claire. "It was like, Oh shit, maybe it's not me, but just what happens when we produce an embryo, the surrogacy route isn't going to work." The news "sent me off the deep end, literally," says Frank. "The hardest thing was I really did see that as my daughter." Frank started to cry. "I was so in love with her. It was amazing for me how strong I felt about something that didn't even exist. I felt this unbelievable love bond of affection for this embryo. When it died, I really felt a part of me died." At Claire's suggestion, Frank went to see a counselor to help him through his grief.

The surrogate wanted to give it another go. To up the odds, the couple did not want to use the frozen embryos, so the doctor harvested another eighteen eggs from Claire, and in February 2000 transferred five fresh embryos to the surrogate. Although hCG levels at first indicated an implantation, none took. The physicians knew that the couple had bonded with this surrogate but encouraged Claire and Frank to try a different one if they still wanted to pursue this avenue.

Frank had given up, but Claire, being Claire, wanted to try the next option on the list. After several months of searching, they found a new surrogate whom Claire felt comfortable with, though Frank did not. They successfully thawed and transferred five of their frozen embryos in August 2000. Again, nothing. A few months later, right before another planned transfer, the surrogate informed them that one of her children had become increasingly uncomfortable about her carrying someone else's baby. "She decided to quit, which was fine with us," said Frank.

In January 2001, Frank learned that his insurance changed its policy and soon would no longer reimburse for fertility problems. Doctors hurriedly harvested another batch of sixteen eggs from Claire, freezing away all of the embryos. A few months later, Frank and Claire met a potential surrogate and her family at Disneyland. They hit it off, and the next month Claire and Frank attended a birthday party for one of the surrogate's three children. "It was building good karma," said Frank.

In June 2001, the clinic accidentally thawed the embryos earlier than planned, and the surrogate had to rush in for a transfer of six embryos that survived the process. "We were all incredibly angry," said Claire. "We figured they had blown our last chance. My body couldn't withstand any more egg retrievals, and we didn't have any more money for it. Economically, psychologically, and physically we were worn out by the process."

They had planned a trip to Paris later that month for Claire's fortieth birthday. On the very day of her birthday, Claire checked her voicemail back in the States, which had a message from the surrogate. She was pregnant. "I knew this one was going to work," said Claire, but, worried about raising Frank's hopes, she decided not to tell him.

An ultrasound showed that the surrogate initially carried twins, but one, in the language of reproduction, vanished.

When the surrogate was four months pregnant, Claire began to feel odd. "I was having hot flashes and thought I was going through menopause," she recalled. "Frank kept saying, 'I bet you you're pregnant, I bet you you're pregnant.'"

Claire, without Frank's knowledge, did a urine test, and when it turned positive she went in for a blood test. The hCG levels came back strong, but she had a grueling business trip to go on and still wanted to wait before breaking the news to him. When she returned, right before Halloween 2001, she told him. "She sat down on the couch and gave me one of those looks that wives give husbands when they have something to say."

"Guess what?" Claire asked.

"You're pregnant," he said straightaway.

"Yep."

"What are we going to do?" Frank asked.

"Nothing," she said.

"Good," he replied.

At the first ultrasound, the doctor found two embryos, but detected a heartbeat from only one. Claire, too, had a vanishing twin.

So now both the surrogate and Claire had viable pregnancies. "I thought, well, here are these twin untwins," said Claire.

Frank went with Claire to the second ultrasound, and as the doctor searched for a beating heart with the Doppler, they expected the worst. The heartbeat thumped, and the doctor turned the volume up.

"Who's your obstetrician?" she asked.

"Obstetrician?" said Claire. "We don't need an obstetrician. It's going to die."

"You come to me one more time, you're going to need a baby doctor," her fertility specialist said.

At the third visit, shortly before Thanksgiving 2001, they returned. The heart continued to beat. "I never in my wildest dreams thought Claire would be pregnant," said Frank. "Part of it was she was convinced that if she had positive thoughts, she would wreck it. Therefore, she would chastise me at every turn any time I was thinking positively."

At week seventeen or so, they considered telling other people, including her father and stepmother, who were planning to come for Christmas. "We're just going to tell them I'm fat," said Claire. "Well, the best-laid plans," said Frank. "You can't hide the fact that there's an elephant in the corner."

They also told their surrogate. Claire and the pregnant surrogate decided to take photos of their two bellies whenever they rendezvoused. "I was really excited, but I kept saying to myself, At least I know this other child is going to work out," said Claire. "This was just the bonus. I was not emotionally attached."

In February 2002, the surrogate's water broke, and Claire and Frank drove the two hours to her hometown to join her for the birth. "It was an odd, surreal scene to watch the birth of our daughter while Claire was five months pregnant," said Frank.

That June, Claire gave birth to a healthy baby boy.

Claire and Frank remain close to the surrogate mother of their daughter to this day. When curious strangers inquire about their two kids, who are four months apart in age, they typically just say they are twins.

In the end, Claire had five miscarriages, fifty-three eggs aspirated from her ovaries, hundreds of blood draws, and white blood cells repeatedly injected into her. A grand total of twenty-six embryos fertilized with Frank's sperm took six separate journeys into the bodies of three different surrogates. I asked both Claire and Frank what they learned from their wild reproductive ride. "With doctors, while they profess to know everything out there, in the fertility world, about one-third of things that go on they can predict, about one-third is educated guessing, and about one-third they have no idea and can't tell you why it happened and whether it will happen again," said Frank. "And that's the sweet spot for the magic of conception and birth." Frank also emphasized to me that he would not choose to do it this way, but he said he would do it again tomorrow. "I consider us the luckiest people in the world."

Claire put markedly more stock in her faith. "I didn't understand what God's plan was for me, but I gave up the control issue," said Claire. "I always felt like it was a deck of cards and they were shuffled. I was dealt a pretty difficult hand for a long time. But when I was given these two gifts — they're both miracles — it was so overpowering. God took away, but gave."

Shannon and I never discussed having a third child. After Ryan arrived, she went on birth control pills and suggested that I have a vasectomy, as several of my friends had done. One friend described the procedure in some detail for me, saying he had trouble walking for a few days and sex did not interest him for weeks afterward. Others insisted that it hardly fazed them. With what Shannon had put her body through for our babies, I did not bother to make the case against vasectomy with her, but the squeamish side of my nature won over the manly man, and I conveniently forgot to make an appointment with the testicle butcher.

Shannon had recurrent migraines, and shortly before the Christmas and Hanukkah holidays in 2001 I went with her to see a neurologist who suspected the birth control pills as the cause. Shannon desperately wanted to avoid migraines during the holidays, so she stopped her pills.

On Valentine's Day 2002, to our astonishment, Shannon and I once again found ourselves debating whether we should waste $10 on a home pregnancy test. Shannon, about to turn forty-four, had not had her period in two weeks, but she had had a rough few weeks at work. She just wanted to enjoy the day, uncomplicated by the pregnancy-miscarriage juggernaut. We had settled into a routine with Ryan, eighteen months old, and Erin, who would turn twelve that May. Life was good. We had demolished our two-bedroom, one-bath house and moved into a rental around the block while we built a new home that could accommodate the four of us.

We bought a pee stick the next day, and sat on our bed and stared in disbelief as it turned positive. We then had a good, long laugh. "It was so absurd," said Shannon. "We knew and expected a miscarriage because we had had miscarriages more times than we had had children," Shannon remembered. Both of us remained completely in denial, and Shannon did not schedule a doctor's appointment until a full month later. Sans a heartbeat, neither of us wanted to invest an emotional cent.

As it happened, Shannon had her first appointment when I was across the country, away at work. I had my cell phone with me, and she promised to phone the minute she learned our fate. By the time I had boarded my plane for the return flight home to San Diego, I had not heard from her. Then, as a flight attendant began to close the door, my phone rang. With another flight attendant walking up the aisle to do whatever it is they do during a crosscheck, I answered my phone. "Yes!" she yelled. "Yes?" I said. The flight attendant gave me that schoolmarmish flight-attendant look. "Yes! Yes! Yes! Yes! Viable! Nine weeks, one day. Cleared for takeoff!" And with that, I said a quick good-bye and hung up. "My wife's pregnant," I blurted out, giddy. So much for keeping my emotions in check.

The pregnancy progressed without a hitch. At thirty-nine weeks, Shannon would have a scheduled C-section on a Monday morning, and she had decided that because the doctors already would have her open, she might as well have her tubes tied. The night of Saturday, October 12, her uterus rumbled, and we drove to the hospital.

Near midnight, the doctors wheeled Shannon into the operating room for a C-section but told me to wait outside until they had given her a spinal anesthetic. I soon heard a scream coming from the direction of the operating room that sounded louder than any woman's scream in the labor and delivery ward. I heard several more before the doctor came out to speak with me. They had tried half a dozen times to inject the spinal, but they could not manage to push the needle in deep enough. With her consent, he explained, they decided to knock Shannon out with a general anesthetic, which pregnant women rarely receive today because it presents more risk to both mother and baby. I no longer was welcome to observe the birth, he said, because Shannon would not be conscious, and the hospital allowed fathers in only if they can offer emotional support.

I just wanted a healthy wife and baby.

Before they placed the anesthesia mask on Shannon's face, she repeatedly told them, "Don't forget the tubes."

Like some scene from a 1940s movie, I paced outside the swinging doors that led to the operating room for what seemed like hours. Finally, the doctor came out and removed his mask. At 2:36 A.M. on October 13, 2004, Shannon gave birth to an eight-pound, twelve-ounce boy, whom we named Aidan Patrick.

"Want to see something interesting?" the doctor asked me.

Before I could answer, he held up a small plastic container filled with pink fluid and toothpick-sized pieces of tissue. "That's from your wife's tubal ligation," he said. I took a long look at this graphic punctuation mark to our reproductive years.

Minutes later, they rolled out my red-faced, smooshed son, and I followed as they pushed him down the hall and into the Neonatal Intensive Care Unit for a short observation period.

And so ended our years of making babies, losing four, but keeping three wondrous, spectacular additions to our life that are nothing short of, yes, miraculous.

I asked Shannon what she made of all this: of having four miscarriages, abandoning the pursuit of more children, becoming pregnant and giving birth at forty-two, going on birth control, briefly going off birth control, and becoming pregnant and giving birth at forty-four. "I think it's random," she said.

When I asked her the same question again the next day, her reply echoed the one I had heard from Claire. "I don't have a whole lot of control over things," Shannon said. "But I have hope. When you have a professional tell you that your chance of carrying to term is less than 3 percent, it's pretty bleak. And then to have two viable pregnancies was life-affirming in every sense of the word."

Miscarriage upended my life. But like Shannon, Claire, Frank, and so many other men and women I met who lose an embryo or a fetus, I, too, gave up control. I, too, accepted my hand. I, too, found my own way of coming to terms with our reproductive limits, only to have fate get the last laugh.

ACKNOWLEDGMENTS

NOTES

GLOSSARY

INDEX

ACKNOWLEDGMENTS

I COULD NOT HAVE WRITTEN THIS BOOK WITHOUT THE SPECTACULAR cooperation I received from women and their partners who have experienced miscarriages. With a few exceptions, these people did not know me, and yet they recounted in terrific detail and typically with tremendous candor some of the most difficult, painful experiences of their lives. They did so, by and large, for the same reason: they wanted their stories to help others caught in the maze of miscarriage, reflecting the special sense of camaraderie that women share with one another. Their club obviously does not include me, which made their enthusiasm for my project that much more striking. I do not have the space to thank them by name, but I deeply appreciate each person's cooperation, and I hope the book serves the purpose they envisioned. I also want to single out the many women and men I spoke with whose stories did not appear here. Each person I interviewed, in some way or another, informed my view of miscarriage. The experiences I chose to recount do not have any more importance than the ones I left out; they simply offered the most compelling illustrations of the scientific questions I chose to explore.

Because I wanted this book to weave together the personal with the scientific, I owe an equal debt to the many clinicians and scientists who generously shared their thoughts with me, allowing me to observe them at work in their laboratories and clinics, answering with extraordinary patience my pestering barrage of e-mails and phone calls, and sending me copies of their hard-to-find studies. On the clinical front, I owe particular thanks to Danny Schust at Boston's Brigham and Women's Hospital, who let me play fly-on-the-wall as he met with his patients. Mary Stephenson and her chief nurse, Edwina Houlihan, repeatedly went out of their way to help me meet patients who came to their Recurrent Pregnancy Loss Clinic located at the Children and Women's Health Centre of British Columbia, Vancouver, Canada. Similarly, the staff at the Recurrent Miscarriage Clinic at St. Mary's Hospital in London, England, allowed me to hang out there and watch its work for the better part of a week, where I met several of the patients whose stories I ended up recounting. Lesley Regan, the head of the clinic, always made me feel welcome and indulged my blend of abundant curiosity and ignorance, as did Raj Rai, May Backos, Jan Brosens, and Safaa El Gaddal. Thanks also goes to their support staff, especially their clinic coordinator, Yvette Fenton.

Many other clinicians who spoke with me at length about their work also made introductions to patients and participants in their clinical studies who shared their stories. I much appreciate the help I received from Alan Beer, E. Nigel Harris, Bruce Lessey, Kypros Nicolaides, and Allen Wilcox.

In my attempt to learn the nuances of reproductive biology and miscarriage, I relied on many tutors and mentors. Each scientist I quote in the book falls into that category, but again, I cannot name them all. Instead, I want to single out a few who either went to extraordinary lengths on my behalf, or who receive no mention elsewhere. From the outset, Kurt Benirschke encouraged me, issued reading assignments (including loans of rare volumes from his library), offered much-welcomed criticisms of my shakier ideas, and allowed me to probe the vast warehouse of knowledge that his mind has accrued about these fields. Kurt also invited me to join him at lectures, private conferences, and autopsies. His guidance proved invaluable, and my gratitude runs deep. I owe a special thanks to Florence Haseltine, who gave me the lay of the land before I had journeyed into this world and connected me to many leading researchers. Vivienne Souter early on helped me shape my thoughts and allowed me to copy her entire library of miscarriage papers. Wendy Robinson made a point of welcoming me to an excellent, invitation-only meeting she organized on genes, chromosomes, and reproduction. Others who assisted my home schooling or made introductions on my behalf but do not appear in these pages include Deborah Anderson, Jacques Cohen, Larry Corey, Ann Duerr, Allen Enders, Gregory Erickson, Barney Graham, Marlys Houck, Joan Hunt, Michael Kettel, Philippe Lazar, Santiago Munné, Tony Plant, Stanley Plotkin, Stephanie Sherman, Keiko Shimizu, Catherine Vandevoort, Linda Van Elsacker, Yury Verlinsky, and Martin Walker.

Several organizations and institutions assisted me. The European Society for Human Reproduction and Embryology allowed me to attend, at no charge, its annual meeting. The Wellcome Library for the History and Understanding of Medicine copied and sent me its entire file on Aleck Bourne. The Biomedical Library at the University of California at San Diego covered most all of my needs for scientific journals and books. Babycenter.com allowed me to post messages in its chatrooms which described my project and led me to several women who had interesting miscarriage stories.

Editors at several magazines supported various aspects of this work. Thanks to Colin Norman, Laura Helmuth, and Leslie Roberts at *Science*; Amy Meeker and Cullen Murphy at the *Atlantic Monthly*; and Rebecca Zacks, Alexandra Stikeman, and David Rotman at *Technology Review*.

As heavily as any book project relies on the kindness of strangers, it needs help from friends and family, too, and many of mine have lent a hand in ways large and small. In a marathon, stress-free editing session, Jack Shafer went through the manuscript with me, helping to excise needless verbiage and passages, fix illogical explanations, and sharpen the focus. I cannot thank him enough. My gratitude also extends to my uncle Larry Kussin, cousins David Kussin and Jeff Daniels, as well as to Edie Munk for her long-standing support.

A few technical details need clarification. Given the sensitive nature of miscarriage and the many privacy issues it raises, I asked all those I spoke with whether they felt comfortable with my using their full names. If they did not, we arrived at a more discreet designation. I did not make up or create any names. Rather, I used people's initials, middle names, or nicknames, noting as much in the text. I hope this strategy both retained the degree of anonymity they sought, yet also did not compromise accuracy or authenticity.

Kurt Benirschke closely read a draft of this book for accuracy, and I thank him for his insightful criticisms. Similarly, Sandra Ann Carson, who graciously agreed to write the foreword for the book, caught many embarrassing mistakes, and I greatly appreciate her input. I was free to ignore their comments, and I, of course, am responsible for all errors.

My editor at Houghton Mifflin, Laura van Dam, had an unwavering commitment to this project and a clearheaded sense of how to make the book as accessible as possible. I thank her for the smart directions and frank judgments she provided, as well as for her patience, an attribute that books uniquely test. Laura's assistant, Erica Avery, also expertly kept the editorial wheels turning. Jayne Yaffe Kemp, the manuscript editor, has one of the finest-toothed combs in the business, as well as a wonderfully sensitive meter for detecting inconsistencies, sloppy logic, and imprecision. Many, many thanks. And thanks to editors Amanda Cook and Wendy Lazear for carrying the book over the finish line.

Gail Ross, my agent, once again offered astute guidance all the way from the birth of the idea through labor and delivery.

I owe a special debt to my parents, Avshalom and Esther Cohen, who not only brought me here and taught me the meaning of family, but also make a point of nourishing my ambitions.

Authors often thank their children for the sacrifices a book project has asked them to make, but that does not apply here. Erin, Ryan, and Aidan made this book possible on a different level altogether. Had I not thoroughly thrilled to Erin joining our lives, the struggle to have more children would not have occurred. Had the struggle to have Ryan not taken place, I doubt that my fascination with miscarriage would have taken root. And had Aidan not magically appeared, how would I have ended my last chapter? So, although not by design, they shaped this project from beginning to end and continue to make my life richer and more fulfilled than I could ever appropriately acknowledge.

My last thank-you, and by all means the most important one, goes to my wife, Shannon. Because of her experience, she served as my guide throughout the research and writing of this book, the authority I repeatedly turned to for counsel, criticism, brainstorming, encouragement, and reality checks. As an extra benefit, Shannon, too, works as a journalist and read and reread my many drafts, catching hundreds of errors and oversights, helping me set a proper tone and pace, and mercilessly redlining passages that altogether needed rethinking. Just as the Lorax in Dr. Seuss spoke for the trees, Shannon spoke for women who miscarried, imploring me to address specific questions that I had not thought of on my own and steering me clear of scientific details she found arcane.

Shannon courageously allowed me to tell, in great detail, her story, too. Her aim had the same altruistic zeal I found in the other women and men I interviewed for this book—and then some. Miscarriage cost her dearly, in a physical and emotional currency that I, as a man, could not possibly experience. Because of this, and the mixture of her good nature and our extraordinary reproductive fate, a passion grew inside of her for this book to come to life. No writer ever could ask for more support from a spouse than that, and it deepened my love and respect for my best friend and partner, with whom, babies or no babies on board, I would want to do it all over again.

NOTES

1: NOT VIABLE

7 Clomid (Clomiphene citrate): Drugs have chemical names when they are under development, generic names (often the same) once they come to market, and then brand names given by each manufacturer. I typically use generic names unless the brand name, like Clomid, is better known. I sometimes use brand names when significant differences exist between products that share a generic name. (Drugs known as human menopausal gonadotropins, for example, can contain different ratios of follicle-stimulating hormone and luteinizing hormone.)

2: THROUGH A GLASS, CLEARLY

23 ovaries removed from fifty-six fetuses: Terry G. Baker, "A Quantitative and Cytological Study of Germ Cells in Human Ovaries," *Proceedings of the Royal Society, Section B, Biological Sciences* 158 (1963): 417–33.

23 utterly convincing paper: In 2004, *Nature* published a study from a team led by Jonathan Tilly at Massachusetts General Hospital that challenged the dogma, providing intriguing evidence that mice continue to generate some eggs into young adulthood. Some scientists immediately hailed the paper as revolutionary, but others cautioned that they wanted to keep their enthusiasm in check until an independent group confirmed the findings. More importantly, no one had yet found similar evidence in humans. See Joshua Johnson, Jacqueline Canning, Tomoko Kaneko, et al., "Germline Stem Cells and Follicular Renewal in the Postnatal Mammalian Ovary," *Nature* 428 (March 11, 2004):

145–50. Allan C. Spradling of the Carnegie Institution of Washington wrote an accompanying editorial in the same issue (133–34). See also Rick Weiss, "Study Casts Doubts on Limits to Fertility," *Washington Post*, March 11, 2004, p. A1.

25   "Both Rock and Hertig": Loretta McLaughlin, *The Pill, John Rock, and the Church: The Biography of a Revolution* (Boston: Little Brown and Company, 1982).

25   During the sixteen years: Arthur T. Hertig, John Rock, Eleanor C. Adams, and William J. Mulligan, "On the Preimplantation Stages of the Human Ovum: A Description of Four Normal and Four Abnormal Specimens Ranging from the Second to the Fifth Day of Development," *Contributions to Embryology* 240 (October 5, 1954): 199–220. Arthur T. Hertig, John Rock, and Eleanor C. Adams, "A Description of 34 Human Ova within the First 17 Days of Development," *American Journal of Anatomy* 98 (May 1956): 435–65.

27   "In a general vein": Arthur Hertig, *Human Trophoblast* (Springfield, Ill.: Charles C. Thomas, 1968).

30   Belgium team of scientists: Jean Schaaps and Jean Hustin made this discovery. See Jean Hustin and Jean P. Schaaps, "Echographic and Anatomic Studies of the Maternotrophoblastic Border during the First Trimester of Pregnancy," *American Journal of Obstetrics and Gynecology* 157 (1987): 162–68; and Jean P. Schaaps and Jean Hustin, "In Vivo Aspect of the Maternal-Trophoblastic Border during the First Trimester of Gestation," *Trophoblast Research* 3 (1998): 39–48.

30   Building on this finding: Graham J. Burton, Eric Jauniaux, and Adrian L. Watson, "Maternal Arterial Connections to the Placental Intervillous Space during the First Trimester of Human Pregnancy: The Boyd Collection Revisited," *American Journal of Obstetrics and Gynecology* 181 (September 1999): 718–24. Graham J. Burton, Adrian L. Watson, Joanne Hempstock, et al., "Uterine Glands Provide Histiotrophic Nutrition for the Human Fetus during the First Trimester of Pregnancy," *Journal of Clinical Endocrinology and Metabolism* 87 (June 2002): 2954–59. Natalie Greenwold, Eric Jauniaux, Beatrice Gulbis, et al., "Relationship among Maternal Serum Endocrinology, Placental Karyotype, and Intervillous Circulation in Early Pregnancy Failure," *Fertility and Sterility* 79 (June 2003): 1373–79.

30   "play a more major role": Don McKay, working with Arthur Hertig and John Rock, actually reported in 1958 that trophoblasts begin incorporating nutrients by the thirteenth day after conception. Arthur Hertig, Eleanor C. Adams, Don McKay, et al., "A Thirteen-Day Human Ovum Studied Histochemically," *American Journal of Obstetrics and Gynecology* 76 (1958): 1025–43.

32   a tiny 0.3 percent: Interestingly, the clinically diagnosed rate of three or more consecutive losses is about 1 percent—still low, but three times higher than predicted by chance alone—which has led many researchers to conclude that

some couples have an increased risk of repeated losses, rather than "consecutive episodes of bad luck," as Lesley Regan and Raj Rai wrote in "Epidemiology and the Medical Causes of Miscarriage," *Baillière's Clinical Obstetrics and Gynaecology* 14 (2000): 839–54. This finding in part justifies the intensified search for medical interventions to help these couples. See also Christine L. Cook and Dwight D. Pridham, "Recurrent Pregnancy Loss," *Current Opinion in Obstetrics and Gynecology* 7 (1995): 357–66.

32 at least half of all conceptions fail: One authoritative estimate concludes that miscarriages occur with 70 percent of conceptions. See Morton A. Stenchever, William Droegemueller, Arthur Herbst, and Daniel Mishell, *Comprehensive Gynecology*, 4th Edition (St. Louis: Mosby, 2001), p. 414.

33 a 1988 issue of the *New England Journal of Medicine*: Allen J. Wilcox, Clarice R. Weinberg, John F. O'Connor, et al., "Incidence of Early Loss of Pregnancy," *New England Journal of Medicine* 319 (July 28, 1988): 189–94.

33 inside that six-day window: Allen J. Wilcox, Clarice R. Weinberg, and Donna Day Baird, "Timing of Sexual Intercourse in Relation to Ovulation," *New England Journal of Medicine* 333 (December 7, 1995): 1517–21.

34 Wilcox's third *New England Journal* article: Allen J. Wilcox, Donna Day Baird, and Clarice R. Weinberg, "Time of Implantation of the Conceptus and Loss of Pregnancy," *New England Journal of Medicine* 340 (June 10, 1999): 1796–99.

3: SCRAMBLED EGGS

37 A 1956 study proved: For a detailed history of human cytogenetics, see James A. Houghton, "Techniques for the Identification of Human Chromosomes," *Scientific Progress* 61 (1974): 461–72.

38 By 1963, both had published evidence: See Thomas M. Clendenin and Kurt Benirschke, "Chromosome Studies on Spontaneous Abortions," *Laboratory Investigations* 12 (1963): 1281–92. Also see David H. Carr, "Chromosome Studies in Abortuses and Stillborn Infants," *Lancet* 2 (September 21, 1963): 603–606. Carr soon became the leading researcher in this field, and by 1966 he had analyzed 227 spontaneous abortions. David H. Carr, "Chromosome Anomalies as a Cause of Spontaneous Abortion," *American Journal of Obstetrics and Gynecology* 97 (1967): 283–93.

38 a mind-stretching *Lancet* article: C. J. Roberts and C. R. Lowe, "Where Have All the Conceptions Gone?" *Lancet* 1 (March 1, 1975): 498–99.

39 first hard evidence that miscarriage occurred much more frequently: Joëlle Boué, André Boué, and Philippe Lazar, "Retrospective and Prospective Epidemiological Studies of 1500 Karyotyped Spontaneous Human Abortions," *Teratology* 12 (1975): 11–26.

39 ob-gyns throughout Paris: The Boués at first collected specimens from hospitals, they explained to me, but they switched to contacting ob-gyns directly because they became concerned that many of their samples came from induced abortions. David Carr told me that he had the same concern about his early data. As Carr explained, because abortion remained illegal at the time he conducted his studies "it was common for people coming into hospital to have abortions that were disguised as miscarriages." Induced abortions, by definition, are of viable pregnancies, and thus would rarely have chromosomal abnormalities. So including them in a study that assessed the frequency of chromosomal aberrations would lower the overall percent of problems detected.

40 chromosomally abnormal embryos typically die shortly after conception: The only trisomies that make it to term involve the sex chromosomes, X and Y, or chromosomes 13, 18, and 21. Monosomies all miscarry, with the exception of the occasional survival of Xo, which leads to a sterile female with what's called Turner syndrome. The rare triploid or tetraploid babies that do not miscarry typically die within a few hours of birth. No one knows precisely why those select chromosomal abnormalities survive, although it may be because they contain fewer genes and play a less critical role in the development of a viable fetus.

41 a richly detailed study of the chromosomes from one thousand miscarriages: Terry Hassold, et al., "A Cytogenetic Study of 1000 Spontaneous Abortions," *Annals of Human Genetics* 44 (1980): 151–64.

42 she analyzed the chromosomes of a man with Klinefelter: Patricia Jacobs and John A. Strong, "A case of human intersexuality having possible XXY sex-determining mechanism," *Nature* 2 (1959): 164–67.

45 harvested eggs from women who had hysterectomies: Kimberly Volarcik, Leon Sheean, James Goldfarb, et al., "The Meiotic Competence of In-Vitro Matured Human Oocytes Is Influenced by Donor Age: Evidence That Folliculogenesis Is Compromised in the Reproductively Aged Ovary," *Human Reproduction*, 13 (1998): 154–60. Another group did similar studies with eggs removed for in vitro fertilization, but those women had taken hormones to induce ovulation, which may themselves influence aneuploidy rates. See David E. Battaglia, P. Goodwin, Nancy A. Klein, et al., "Influence of Maternal Age on Meiotic Spindle Assembly in Oocytes from Natural Cycling Women," *Human Reproduction* 11 (1996): 2217–22.

46 a most unusual assertion about chromosomal sex: S. Alan Henderson and Robert G. Edwards, "Chiasma Frequency and Maternal Age in Mammals," *Nature* 218 (April 6, 1968): 22–28.

46 fly geneticists studied the X chromosome: Kara E. Koehler et al., "Spontaneous X Chromosome MI and MII Nondisjunction Events in *Drosophila melanogaster*

Oocytes Have Different Recombinational Histories," *Nature Genetics* 14 (December 1996): 406–13.

46   examined Down syndrome in people: Neil E. Lamb et al., "Susceptible Chiasmate Configurations of Chromosome 21 Predispose to Non-disjunction in Both Maternal Meiosis I and Meiosis II," *Nature Genetics* 14 (December 1996): 400–405.

47   Hogge conducted his own cost-effectiveness study: See W. Alan Hogge, A. L. Byrnes, M. C. Lanasa, et al., "The Clinical Use of Karyotyping Spontaneous Abortions," *American Journal of Obstetrics and Gynecology* 189 (August 2003): 397–400. An early study by investigators at the University of South Carolina had addressed the same question and also found a cost benefit. Gordon C. Wolf and Edgar O. Horger, "Indications for Examination of Spontaneous Abortion Specimens: A Reassessment," *American Journal of Obstetrics and Gynecology*, 173 (November 1995): 1364–68.

48   went up to only 16 percent: U. B Knudsen, V. Hansen, S. Juul, et al., "Prognosis of a New Pregnancy Following Previous Spontaneous Abortions," *European Journal of Obstetrics & Gynecology and Reproductive Biology* 39 (1991): 31–36.

48   201 women who had no identified underlying problem: Katy Clifford, Raj Rai, and Lesley Regan, "Future Pregnancy Outcome in Unexplained Recurrent First Trimester Miscarriage," *Human Reproduction* 12 (February 1997): 387–89.

48   age matters more than miscarriage history: Roy Farquharson and his coworkers at Liverpool Women's Hospital reviewed patient information from 716 patients who attended the miscarriage clinic there. Of the 226 who conceived and had no determined underlying problem, 75 percent carried to term. The researchers further divided the women who had losses both by how many previous miscarriages they had and by their age. Age increased a woman's risk more than her miscarriage history, which a telling table illustrated: At twenty, a woman with four previous losses had a 12 percent chance of miscarrying; at forty, the miscarriage rate in a woman with the same history jumped to 32 percent. "A Longitudinal Study of Pregnancy Outcome Following Idiopathic Recurrent Miscarriage," *Human Reproduction* 14 (1999): 2868–71.

50   new method adopted from cancer research: Anne Kallioniemi, Olli-P. Kallioniemi, Damir Sudar, et al., "Comparative Genomic Hybridization for Molecular Cytogenetic Analysis of Solid Tumors," *Science* 258 (October 30, 1992): 818–21.

51   comparative genomic hybridization could affect miscarriage: Brenda Lomax, Steven Tang, Evica Separovic, et al., "Comparative Genomic Hybridization in Combination with Flow Cytometery Improves Results of Cytogenetic Analysis of Spontaneous Abortions," *American Journal of Human Genetics* 66 (2000): 1561–21.

51   Malpas recognized this dilemma: Percy Malpas, "A Study of Abortion Sequences," *Journal of Obstetrics and Gynaecology of the British Empire* 45 (1938): 932–49.

52   which informed the medical community for decades: In 1956, Nicholson J. Eastman wrote a chapter for the popular medical textbook *Williams' Obstetrics*, which showed how his own calculations supported Malpas's findings—with an astonishing 84 percent of women who miscarried three times destined to lose their fourth pregnancies. Dorothy Warburton and F. Clarke Fraser of McGill University in Montreal finally refuted Malpas and Eastman in a classic 1961 paper that exposed the flawed logic of their predecessors. See Nicholson J. Eastman, *Williams' Obstetrics*, 11th edition, Chapter 21, New York: Appleton-Century-Crofts. See also Dorothy Warburton and F. Clarke Fraser, "On the Probability That a Woman Who Has Had a Spontaneous Abortion Will Abort in Subsequent Pregnancies," *Journal of Obstetrics and Gynaecology of the British Commonwealth* 68 (1961): 784–87.

52   underscored how much diversity exists: Mary D. Stephenson, Khalid A. Awartani, and Wendy P. Robinson, "Cytogenetic Analysis of Miscarriages from Couples with Recurrent Miscarriage: A Case-Control Study," *Human Reproduction* 17 (February 2002): 446–51.

4: REJECTION

58   lymphocyte immune therapy: This intervention has many other names, including paternal cell, mononuclear cell, or leukocyte immunization.

59   dates back to 1952: Peter B. Medawar, "Some Immunological and Endocrinological Problems Raised by the Evolution of Viviparity in Vertebrates," *Symposia of the Society for Experimental Biology* 7 (1953): 320–28.

60   bar codes to distinguish self from nonself: A variety of human leukocyte antigens, first described in 1958 by France's Jean Dausset (he won the Nobel Prize in 1980 for the discovery), make up this bar code system. See Jean Dausset, "Iso-leuco-anticorps," *Acta Hematologica* 20 (1958): 156–66, and his Nobel Prize lecture, "The Major Histocompatibility Complex in Man," *Science* 213 (September 25, 1981): 1469–74.

61   In a two-part paper: Rupert E. Billingham, "Transplantation Immunity and the Maternal-Fetal Relation," *New England Journal of Medicine* 270 (March 26 and April 2, 1964): 667–72 and 720–25.

62   In 1973, *Science* published: Alan E. Beer and Rupert E. Billingham, "Maternally Acquired Runt Disease: Immune Lymphocytes from the Maternal Blood Can Traverse the Placenta and Cause Runt Disease in the Progeny," *Science* 4070 (January 19, 1973): 240–43.

62   journals as discriminating as *Science:* When I speak of *Science* as "discriminating," I am referring to the peer-reviewed, scientific papers that describe new data. I write for the news department of *Science*, and while I believe my editors have the highest standards and certainly hope our stories have impact, they do not go through a peer review.

62   ran in the widely read *Scientific American:* Alan E. Beer and Rupert E. Billingham, "The Embryo as a Transplant," *Scientific American* 230 (April 1974): 36–46.

64   a paper describing her case: Alan E. Beer et al., "Major Histocompatibility Complex Antigens, Maternal and Paternal Immune Responses, and Chronic Habitual Abortions in Humans," *American Journal of Obstetrics and Gynecology* 141 (December 15, 1981): 987–99.

66   A 1986 story in *Newsweek:* Jerry Adler et al., "Learning from the Loss," *Newsweek* (March 24, 1986): 66.

69   had spread worldwide: Peter Castro and Giovanna Breu, "Injection of Hope," *People* (October 28, 1996), and Bob Arnot, "The New Frontier," *Dateline* NBC (December 18, 2000).

71   a most cordial note: Beer's tone markedly changed as I delved more deeply into the scientific issues. After my calls to the Food and Drug Administration about lymphocyte immune therapy apparently led the FDA to contact Beer, he questioned whether I had misrepresented his work to the agency—which I had not —and he signed off with this warning: "MY LEGAL ADVISORS WILL CONTACT YOU."

71   on average, 38.6 years old: Beer referred to the average patient both on his Web site and in an e-mail exchange on June 23, 1999, with women who joined a chat in which he served as a guest speaker on the Web site run by the InterNational Council on Infertility Information Dissemination. In that same discussion, he described a success rate of 86.9 percent for women who have what he refers to as category 1 and category 5 problems and receive treatment before conception. Again, as his Web site explained in detail in July 2001, the treatment for both category 1 (defined as couples with too much genetic similarity) and category 5 problems (elevated natural killer cells and antihormone antibodies) was lymphocyte immune therapy. (He noted that some women with category 5 problems also would require intravenous immunoglobulin.) Beer explained to me that he knew that only 25 percent would succeed without lymphocyte immune therapy because of the several hundred couples he advised to do the treatment who became pregnant before starting it.

75   a bulletin board on the Yahoo Web site: The address for this group, which noted that it works closely with Beer, is http://health.groups.yahoo.com/group/immunologysupport (last accessed July 23, 2004).

76   in 111 Hutterite couples: Carole Ober et al., "Human Leukocyte Antigen Match-

ing and Fetal Loss: Results of a 10-Year Prospective Study," *Human Reproduction* 13 (1998): 33–38. See also Carole Ober, "HLA and Pregnancy: The Paradox of the Fetal Allograft," *American Journal of Human Genetics* 62 (1998): 1–5.

77   with the discovery in 1986: Shirley Ellis et al., "Evidence for a Novel HLA Antigen Found on Human Extravillous Trophoblast and a Choriocarcinoma Cell Line," *Immunology* 59 (December 1986): 595–601. Researchers first tied this "novel HLA antigen" to HLA-G four years later. See Susan Kovats et al., "A Class I Antigen, HLA-G, Expressed in Human Trophoblasts," *Science* 248 (April 13, 1990): 220–23, and Shirley Ellis, M. S. Palmer, and Andrew McMichael, "Human Trophoblast and the Choriocarcinoma Cell Line BeWo, Express a Truncated HLA Class I Molecule," *Journal of Immunology* 144 (1990): 731–35.

77   differs remarkably little: To appreciate the complex interaction between HLA-G and the immune system, see J. LeMaoult et al., "Biology and Functions of Human Leukocyte Antigen-G in Health and Sickness," *Tissue Antigens* 62 (2003): 273–84.

77   HLA-G occupies center stage: Nathalie Rouas-Freiss et al., "Direct Evidence to Support the Role of HLA-G in Protecting the Fetus from Maternal Uterine Natural Killer Cytolysis," *Proceedings of the National Academy of Sciences* 94 (October 1997): 11520–25. Philippe Le Bouteiller et al., "Soluble HLA-G1 at the Materno-Foetal Interface — A Review," *Trophoblast Research* 24, Supplement A (2003): S10–15.

78   Ober, Stephenson, Scott: Carrie Aldrich et al., "HLA-G Genotypes and Pregnancy Outcome in Couples with Recurrent Miscarriage," *Molecular Human Reproduction* 7 (2001): 1167–72.

78   a research group in Germany: K. A. Pfeiffer et al., "The HLA-G Genotype Is Potentially Associated with Idiopathic Recurrent Spontaneous Abortion," *Molecular Human Reproduction* 7 (2001): 373–78.

78   Yet another study: Beatrice Fuzzi et al., "HLA-G Expression in Early Embryos Is a Fundamental Prerequisite for the Obtainment of Pregnancy," *European Journal of Immunology* 32 (2002): 311–15.

78   Contradictory results challenge: David Bainbridge, Shirley Ellis, Philippe Le Bouteiller, and Ian Sargent, "HLA-G Remains a Mystery," *Trends in Immunology* 22 (October 2001): 548–52. See also Radhika N. Patel et al., "Expression of Membrane-bound HLA-G at the Maternal-Fetal Interface Is Not Associated with Pregnancy Maintenance among Patients with Idiopathic Recurrent Miscarriage," *Molecular Human Reproduction* 9 (2003): 551–57.

78   the story of a thirty-seven-year-old corporate attorney: Daniel Wallace and Michael Weisman, "The Use of Etanercept and Other Tumor Necrosis Factor-α Blockers in Infertility: It's Time to Get Serious," *Journal of Rheumatology* 30 (September 2003): 1897–99.

79 This hugely controversial hypothesis: Th1 and Th2 actually refer to the white blood cells, called T-helper cells, that secrete the bulk of the chemical messengers, or cytokines. Timothy Mosmann, Robert Coffman, and colleagues at the DNAX Research Institute first reported the Th1/Th2 dichotomy in mice. See Timothy Mosmann, Holly Cherwinski, Martha W. Bond, et al., "Two Types of Murine Helper T Cell Clone," *Journal of Immunology* 136 (April 1, 1986): 2348–57. Mosmann later teamed up with the University of Alberta's Thomas Wegmann, who long had studied immunoprotection in pregnant mice, and together they postulated that a Th2 state might protect the fetus. See Thomas G. Wegmann, Hui Lin, Larry Guildbert, et al., "Bidirectional Cytokine Interactions in the Maternal-Fetal Relationship: Is Successful Pregnancy a Th2 Phenomenon?" *Immunology Today* 14 (1993): 353–56. Joseph Hill, who for several years ran the Recurrent Miscarriage Clinic at Boston's Brigham and Women's Hospital, subsequently published several studies supporting the theory, including Zhigang C. Wang, Edmond J. Yunis, and Maria J. De los Santos, et al., "T Helper 1-Type Immunity to Trophoblast Antigens in Women with a History of Recurrent Pregnancy Loss Is Associated with Polymorphism of the IL1B Promoter Region," *Genes and Immunity* 3 (2002): 38–42. But other studies have challenged the theory, all of which is covered in a detailed overview by S. M. Laird, E. M. Tuckerman, B. A. Cork, et al., "A Review of Immune Cells and Molecules in Women with Recurrent Miscarriage," *Human Reproduction Update* 9 (2003): 163–74.

5: BLACK SWANS

83 A 1954 paper did link this lupus anticoagulant: Jean-Louis Beaumont, "Syndrome Hémorragique Acquis du à un Anticoagulant Circulant," *Sang* 25 (1954): 1–15.

84 The breakthrough came in 1983: E. Nigel Harris et al., "Anticardiolipin Antibodies: Detection by Radioimmunoassay and Association with Thrombosis in Systemic Lupus Erythematosus," *Lancet*, 2 (November 26, 1983): 1211–14.

84 in one of his many papers: E. Nigel Harris, "Syndrome of the Black Swan," *British Journal of Rheumatology* 26 (1987): 324–26.

86 "immunological Wars of the Roses": Norbert Gleicher, Andrea Vidali, and Vishvanath Karande, "The Immunological 'Wars of the Roses': Disagreements Amongst Reproductive Immunologists," *Human Reproduction* 17 (March 2002): 539–42.

86 Kutteh, a recurrent miscarriage specialist: William Kutteh, "Antiphospholipid Antibody-Associated Recurrent Pregnancy Loss: Treatment with Heparin and Low-Dose Aspirin Is Superior to Low-Dose Aspirin Alone," *American Journal of*

Obstetrics and Gynecology 174 (May 1996): 1584–89. Lesley Regan's group paper appeared six months later. Raj Rai et al., "Randomised Controlled Trial of Aspirin and Aspirin Plus Heparin in Pregnant Women with Recurrent Miscarriage Associated with Phospholipid Antibodies (or Antiphospholipid Antibodies)," *British Medical Journal* 314 (January 25, 1997): 253–57. The accompanying editorial by Munther Khamashta and Charles Mackworth-Young appeared on page 245 of the same issue of the *British Medical Journal*.

86   the world's largest study to assess the frequency: Raj S. Rai, Lesley Regan, Kathy Clifford, et al., "Antiphospholipid antibodies and β2-Glycoprotein-1 in 500 Women with Recurrent Miscarriage: Results of a Comprehensive Screening Approach," *Human Reproduction* 10 (1995): 2001–2005. A smaller study that included only women who had three consecutive miscarriages and no evidence of karyotypically normal abortuses found that 17 percent had antiphospholipid antibody syndrome. See Mary Stephenson, "Frequency of Factors Associated with Habitual Abortion in 197 Couples," *Fertility and Sterility* 66 (July 1996): 24–29. Researchers from the miscarriage clinic at the Liverpool Women's Hospital study of 427 women who had at least two consecutive losses determined that 21 percent either had or possibly had antiphospholipid syndrome. See L. Bricker and R. G. Farquharson, "Types of Pregnancy Loss in Recurrent Miscarriage: Implications for Research and Clinical Practice," *Human Reproduction* 17 (2002): 1345–50.

87   a stunning study: Neil J. Sebire et al., "Defective Endovascular Trophoblast Invasion in Primary Antiphospholipid Antibody Syndrome–Associated Early Pregnancy Failure," *Human Reproduction* 17 (2002): 1067–71.

88   Blood clots, he pointed out: Implantation, as I describe in chapter 2, depends on trophoblasts invading the maternal arteries and briefly plugging them, during which time the trophoblasts convert the flexible walls of the arteries into more rigid pipes that can handle the higher blood flow needed to supply the fetus with oxygen. During this process, the embryo and early fetus need little oxygen and, indeed, too much oxygen in an embryo indicates a failure.

88   The spirited, even contentious, debates: For a flavor of the tenor, see the letters to the editor in the December 2002 *Obstetrics & Gynecology*, pp. 1354–56, written by Lesley Regan and Raj Rai, and, separately, William Kutteh, criticizing a study by Roy Farquharson and colleagues. For skeptical reports of the association between antiphospholipid antibodies and miscarriage, see Sophia Stone et al., "Antiphospholipid Antibodies Do Not a Syndrome Make," *Lupus* 11 (2002): 130–33 and Joe Simpson et al., "Lack of Association Between Antiphospholipid Antibodies and First-Trimester Spontaneous Abortion: Prospective Study of Pregnancies Detected Within 21 Days of Conception," *Fertility and Sterility* 69 (May 1998): 814–20. For an excellent overview of the de-

bates, see D. Ware Branch and Munther Khamashta, "Antiphospholipid Syndrome: Obstetric Diagnosis, Management and Controversies," *Obstetrics & Gynecology* 101 (June 2003): 1333–44. In the same vein, see Caleb Kallen and Aydin Arici, "Immune Testing in Fertility Practice: Truth or Deception," *Current Opinion in Obstetrics and Gynecology* 15 (2003) 225–31.

90   of at least nine inherited blood-clotting problems: In addition to factor V Leiden, others include antithrombin III deficiency, protein C deficiency, protein S deficiency, prothrombin G20210A mutation, dysfibrinogemia, activated protein C resistance, hyperhomocysteinemia, and factor II mutation. Zeev Blumenfeld and Benjamin Brenner offer a thorough review of their links to miscarriage in "Thrombophilia-Associated Pregnancy Wastage," *Fertility and Sterility* 72 (November 1999): 765–74. For an analysis of the strength of the association between several of these disorders and miscarriage, see Evelyne Rey et al., "Thrombopilic Disorders and Fetal Loss: A Meta-analysis," *Lancet* 361 (March 15, 2003): 901–908.

90   Although no rigorous clinical trial: Raj Rai et al., "Factor V Leiden and Recurrent Miscarriages—Prospective Outcome of Untreated Pregnancies," *Human Reproduction* 17 (2002): 442–45. This paper discusses the two clinical studies that had occurred by then.

91   Originally described in 1948: Charles W. Whitten and Philip E. Greilich, "Thromboelastography®: Past, Present, and Future," *Anesthesiology* 92 (2000): 1223–25.

91   The study examined the blood of 494 such women: Raj Rai, Edward Tuddenham, May Backos, et al., "Thromboelastography, Whole-Blood Haemostasis and Recurrent Miscarriage," *Human Reproduction* 18 (December 2003): 2540–43.

92   preeclampsia, a life-threatening high blood pressure: For an authoritative overview of this complication, see Chris Redman and Ian Sargent, "Preeclampsia, the Placenta and the Maternal Systemic Inflammatory Response—A Review," *Placenta* 24, Supplement A (2003): S21–27.

94   So-called intravenous immunoglobulin: The first report in the literature of IVIG used to treat miscarriage came from a research group in Germany. G. Mueller-Eckhardt et al., "Prevention of Recurrent Spontaneous Abortion by Intravenous Immunoglobulin," *Vox Sang* 56 (1989): 151–54.

94   First licensed in 1981: For an overview of IVIG's on- and off-label use, see Peter D. Donofrio and Neil A. Busis, "Regulatory and Reimbursement Issues in Treating Patients with Immune-Mediated Neuropathies," *Neurology* 59, Supplement 6 (December 24, 2002): S41–45.

95   Six small-scale, randomized: James Scott published a meta-analysis of these studies and a seventh one published after Stephenson started her study. After combining the studies, Scott found "no significant increase in the overall preg-

nancy success rate." James R. Scott, "Immunotherapy for Recurrent Miscarriage," Cochrane Library 2 (2004). The Cochrane Library is an online database of "evidence-based" medicine that features meta-analysis, referred to as "systematic reviews."

95 research groups have proposed mechanisms: For an overview of potential IVIG mechanisms, see pp. 628 and 629 of Mary Stephenson and Mary Ensom, "An Update on the Role of Immunotherapy in Reproductive Failure," *Immunology and Allergy Clinics of North America* 22 (2002): 623–42.

95 contaminations occurred: No author, "Epidemiologic Notes and Reports Outbreak of Hepatitis C Associated with Intravenous Immunoglobulin Administration—United States, October 1993–June 1994," *Morbidity and Mortality Weekly Report* 43 (July 22, 1994): 505–509.

6: THE CYCLE OF LIFE

97 Way back in the fourth century: Colin A. Finn, "Why Do Women Menstruate? Historical and Evolutionary Review," *European Journal of Obstetrics and Gynecology* 70 (1996): 3–8.

97 few species menstruate: In addition to primates, fruit bats and elephant shrews menstruate. See Colin A. Finn's earlier paper on the subject, "Why Do Women and Some Other Primates Menstruate?" *Perspectives in Biology and Medicine* 30 (1987): 566–74.

98 "changes from soil into bricks": For an excellent review of trophoblast invasion and menstruation, see Harvey Jon Kliman, "Uteroplacental Blood Flow," *American Journal of Pathology* 157 (December 2000): 1759–68.

98 clear the uterus of pathogens: The *Quarterly Review of Biology*, over five years, published the main menstruation arguments and counterarguments that I discuss. It began with Margie Profet, a recipient of the MacArthur Foundation "genius" award, and the pathogen thesis. Margie Profet, "Menstruation as a Defense Against Pathogens Transported by Sperm," *Quarterly Review of Biology* 68 (September 1993): 335–86. The anthropologist Beverly Strassmann, who famously studied menstruation in the Dogon of Mali, countered with the metabolic energy conservation argument. Beverly I. Strassmann, "The Evolution of Endometrial Cycles and Menstruation," *Quarterly Review of Biology* 71 (June 1996): 181–220. Colin Finn had the last word. Colin A. Finn, "Menstruation: A Nonadaptive Consequence of Uterine Evolution," *Quarterly Review of Biology* 73 (June 1998): 163–73.

99 a "window of implantation" exists: Alexander Psychoyos first proposed the idea a year before Finn, but researchers in the field often cite them in the same breath. Alexander Psychoyos, "Hormonal Control of Ovoimplantation," *Vita-*

mins and Hormones 31 (1973): 201–56. Colin A. Finn and L. Martin, "The Control of Implantation," *Journal of Reproduction and Fertility* 39 (1974): 195–206.

99   potentially life-threatening: The condition in which the trophoblasts bore too deeply has three names — "placenta accreta," "increta," or "percreta" — that delineate, respectively, increasing depths of the abnormal invasion.

99   a deficient luteal phase: As befitting a controversial condition, doctors have used many terms to describe it, including, "luteal phase defect," "luteal insufficiency," "inadequate corpus luteum," "luteal phase inadequacy," "corpus luteum insufficiency," and "corpus luteum dysfunction."

103   sex glands secreted special juices: Julia Ellen Rechter, a graduate student in history at the University of California at Berkeley, wrote a comprehensive analysis of the early days of reproductive endocrinology in her 1997 doctoral dissertation, "'The Glands of Destiny': A History of Popular, Medical and Scientific Views of the Sex Hormones in 1920s America," UMI Number 9827084. See also Jean D. Wilson, "Endocrinology: Survival as a Discipline in the 21st Century?" *Annual Review of Physiology* 62 (2000): 947–50.

104   begins in the nose: Donald Pfaff and Marlene Schwanzel-Fukuda at Rockefeller University first made this astonishing finding in mice and later described it in human embryos. They discuss the mouse studies in Marlene Schwanzel-Fukuda and Donald Pfaff, "Origin of Luteinizing Hormone-Releasing Hormone Neurons," *Nature* 338 (March 9, 1989): 161–64. For the human studies, see Marlene Schwanzel-Fukuda, Kathryn L. Crossin, Donald W. Pfaff, et al., "Migration of Luteinizing Hormone-Releasing Hormone (LHRH) Neurons in Early Human Embryos," *Journal of Comparative Neurology* 366 (March 11, 1996): 547–57.

104   two back-to-back *Science* papers: Ernest Knobil, Tony Plant, Ludwig Wildt, et al., "Control of the Rhesus Monkey Menstrual Cycle: Permissive Role of Hypothalamic Gonoadotropin-Releasing Hormone," *Science* 207 (March 21, 1980): 1371–73, and Ludwig Wildt, Gary Marshall, and Ernest Knobil, "Experimental Induction of Puberty in the Infantile Female Rhesus Monkey," *Science* 207 (March 21, 1980): 1373–75.

104   the onset of puberty: No one knows why puberty starts, but researchers have in the past twenty years unearthed some fascinating clues. The GnRH pulses start in the fetus, yet they have no effect because hormones made by the placenta create biochemical brakes. At about four to five months after birth, the body sends out its own biochemical brakes that shut down production of GnRH. Colorful, beguiling theories have attempted to explain what removes the biological brakes, though at this point, no hypothesis satisfies far beyond the person who has proposed it. Scientists have argued that puberty's onset has to do with everything from "bone age" to the amount of light a child re-

ceives to nutrition and the accumulation of fat and weight. A coauthor of the original work with Knobil has written a thorough overview of the onset of puberty. See Tony Plant, "Neurological Bases Underlying the Control of the Onset of Puberty in the Rhesus Monkey: A Representative Higher Primate," *Frontiers in Neuroendocrinology* 22 (2001): 107–39. For an intriguing look at the light hypothesis, see Leona Zacharias and Richard Wurtman, "Blindness: Its Relation to Age of Menarche," *Science* 144 (May 29, 1964): 1154–55.

106 the hormonal dance begins anew: Complex as this all may seem, I intentionally have grossly *oversimplified* the process of ovulation, which recent research has shown also relies heavily on growth factors supplied by the dominant follicle itself. See Gregory F. Erickson and Shunichi Shimasaki, "The Physiology of Folliculogenesis: The Role of Novel Growth Factors," *Fertility and Sterility* 76 (November 2001): 943–49.

106 Just as luteinizing hormone nourishes the follicle: Luteinizing hormone and human chorionic gonadotropin have similar chemical structures.

106 A bizarre study: Arpad Csapo, Martii O. Pulkkinen, B. Ruttner, et al., "The Significance of the Human Corpus Luteum in Pregnancy Maintenance: Preliminary Studies," *American Journal of Obstetrics and Gynecology* 112 (April 15, 1972): 1061–67.

108 an exhaustive examination: Richmal Marie Oates-Whitehead, David Haas, and Judith Carrier, "Progestogen for Preventing Miscarriage," *Cochrane Library* 4 (2003).

111 the first such massive analysis: Daniel D. Carson, Errin Lagow, Amantha Thathiah, et al., "Changes in Gene Expression During the Early to Mid-luteal (Receptive Phase) Transition in Human Endometrium Detected by High-Density Microarray Screening," *Molecular Human Reproduction* 8 (September 2002): 871–79. Lessey later collaborated with Linda Giudice's team at Stanford University and further identified specific genes potentially involved with implantation failure. Lee-Chuan Kao, Ariane Germeyer, Suzana Tulac, et al., "Expression Profiling of Endometrium from Women with Endometriosis Reveals Candidate Genes for Disease-based Implantation Failure and Infertility," *Endocrinology* 144 (July 2003): 2870–81.

112 including one completely fraudulent one, later retracted: See J. Malcom Pearce and Rosol I. Hamid, "Randomised Controlled Trial of the Use of Human Chorionic Gonadotropin in Recurrent Miscarriage Associated with Polycystic Ovaries," *British Journal of Obstetrics and Gynecology* 101 (August 1994): 685–88. A retraction appeared in the *British Journal of Obstetrics and Gynecology* 102 (November 1995): 853. A November 17, 1994, story in London's *Daily Mail* first reported the fraud allegations against Pearce, which also included a paper published in the same medical journal about an ectopic pregnancy that he

supposedly removed and then successfully implanted through the vagina. See Jenny Hope and Greg Hadfield, "Baby Doctors in Hoax Probe; Cloud Over Operation that Gave Hope to Thousands of Women," *Daily Mail*, November 17, 1994, p. 1.

112 randomly assigned hCG or a placebo: Siobhan Quenby and Roy Farquharson, "Human Chorionic Gonadotropin Supplementation in Recurring Pregnancy Loss: A Controlled Trial," *Fertility and Sterility* 62 (October 1994): 708–10. For a meta-analysis of other hCG/miscarriage studies, see James R. Scott and Neil Pattison, "Human Chorionic Gonadotropin for Recurrent Miscarriage," Cochrane Library 4 (2003).

113 known as polycysts: Polycysts on the ovaries have nothing to do with cancerous cysts.

113 In 1990, Lesley Regan: For a detailed description of polycystic ovaries in a miscarriage clinic, see Raj Rai, May Backos, Frances Rushworth, and Lesley Regan, "Polycystic Ovaries and Recurrent Miscarriage — A Reappraisal," *Human Reproduction* 15 (2000): 612–15. Stephen Franks wrote an excellent overview, "Polycystic Ovary Syndrome," *New England Journal of Medicine* 333 (September 28, 1995): 853–61.

114 Obesity itself: For a review of the link between obesity and miscarriage, see Robert J. Norman and A. M. Clark, "Obesity and Reproductive Disorders, a Review," *Reproduction, Fertility and Development* 10 (1998): 55–63. Norman's group also specifically analyzed the role of obesity and miscarriage in women with PCOS. See Jim X. Wang, Michael J. Davies, and Robert J. Norman, "Polycystic Ovarian Syndrome and the Risk of Spontaneous Abortion Following Assisted Reproduction Technology Treatment," *Human Reproduction* 16 (2001): 2606–609.

114 metformin, which helps the body use insulin: Both of these research groups conclude their reports by calling for a randomized, placebo-controlled study. See Daniela J. Jakubowicz, Maria Iuorno, Salomon Jakubowicz, et al., "Effects of Metformin on Early Pregnancy Loss in the Polycystic Ovary Syndrome," *Journal of Clinical Endocrinology and Metabolism* 87 (February 2002): 524–29. Also see Charles J. Glueck, Ping Wang, Naila Goldenberg et al., "Pregnancy Outcomes Among Women with Polycystic Ovary Syndrome Treated with Metformin," *Human Reproduction* 17 (2002): 2858–64.

114 letrozole, an estrogen-blocking drug: Robert Casper's group at the University of Toronto pioneered this work. See Stephanie A. Fisher, Robert L. Reid, Dean A. Van Vugt, and Robert F. Casper, "A Randomized Double-Blind Comparison of the Effects of Clomiphene Citrate and the Aromatase Inhibitor Letrozole on Ovulatory Function in Normal Women," *Fertility and Sterility* 78 (August 2002): 280–85. Letrozole, which goes by the brand name Femera, inhibits an enzyme

called aromatase, which the body uses to convert male hormones into estro-gen. For a detailed discussion of letrozole's mechanism of action, see Mo-hamed Mitwally and Robert F. Casper, "Aromatase Inhibition for Ovarian Stim-ulation: Future Avenues for Fertility Management," *Current Opinion in Obstetrics and Gynecology* 14 (2002): 255–63.

114   a treatment guideline: "The Investigation and Treatment of Couples with Re-current Miscarriage," Royal College of Obstetricians and Gynaecologists, Guideline No. 17, May 2003.

7: REALLY?

117   In 1969, a mother of one of the girls: Robert Meyers, in his brilliantly detailed book, DES: *The Bitter Pill* (New York: Seaview/Putnam, 1983), recounts how Ulfelder and Herbst first thought to connect the adenocarcinoma cases to DES. See Chapter 7, pp. 93–110. I discussed the passage with Herbst, who confirmed its accuracy.

117   "When I was pregnant with her": This account comes from Robert Meyers, DES: *The Bitter Pill*, New York: Seaview/Putnam, 1983, p. 93.

117   Stilbestrol, a trade name: For a listing of various names used for DES-type drugs, see Table 1 in Barbara Hammes and Cynthia J. Laitman, "Diethyl-stilbestrol (DES) Update: Recommendations for the Identification and Man-agement of DES-Exposed Individuals," *Journal of Midwifery & Women's Health* 48 (2003): 19–29. Laitman also authored DES: *The Complete Story*, St. Martin's Press, 1981.

117   the synthetic estrogen: E. Charles Dodds of the University of London in 1938 first reported the synthesis of diethylstilbestrol, the first estrogen that could be taken as a pill. E. Charles Dodds, L. Goldberg, W. Lawson, and R. Robin-son, "Estrogenic Activity of Certain Synthetic Compounds," *Nature* 141 (1938): 247–48. DES won approval from the U.S. Food and Drug Administration in 1941 to treat gonorrhea, vaginitis, and menopausal symptoms, and to suppress lactation. In 1947, it won FDA approval for treatment in pregnant women. For a detailed description of the approval process, see Roberta J. Apfel and Susan M. Fisher, *To Do No Harm: DES and the Dilemmas of Modern Medicine*, New Haven/London: Yale University Press, 1984, pp. 19 and 20.

118   the little-noticed *Cancer* paper: Arthur L. Herbst and Robert E. Scully, "Adeno-carcinoma of the Vagina in Adolescence," *Cancer* 25 (April 1970): 745–57.

118   Herbst took a copy of their paper: Arthur L. Herbst, Howard Ulfelder, and David C. Poskanzer, "Adenocarcinoma of the Vagina: Association of Maternal Stilbestrol Therapy with Tumor Appearance in Young Women," *New England*

Journal of Medicine 284 (April 22, 1971): 878–81. The editorial by Alexander Langmuir, "New Environmental Factor in Congenital Disease," ran in the same issue, pp. 912–13.

119 had ballooned to the point: "Hormonal Time Bomb? Treatment with Diethylstilbestrol, Cause of Vaginal Cancer," *Time* 98 (August 2, 1971), pp. 52–53. Less than two weeks later, New York public health officials reported their own investigation that linked in utero DES exposure to adenocarcinoma. Peter Greenwald, Joseph Barlow, Philip C. Nasca, et al., "Vaginal Cancer after Maternal Treatment with Synthetic Estrogens," *New England Journal of Medicine* 285 (August 12, 1971): 390–92.

119 in one thirty-six-year-old pregnant woman: Olive Watkins Smith, George Van S. Smith, and David Hurwitz, "Increased Excretion of Pregnanediol in Pregnancy from Diethylstilbestrol with Special Reference to the Prevention of Late Pregnancy Accidents," *American Journal of Obstetrics and Gynecology* 51 (1946): 411–15.

120 Olive Smith presented findings: Smith made her presentation to the Norfolk District Medical Society in Boston, Massachusetts, on February 24, 1948, which appeared later that year as "Diethylstilbestrol in the Prevention and Treatment of Complications of Pregnancy," *American Journal of Obstetrics and Gynecology* 56 (November 1948): 821–34.

121 Smiths reported findings from a controlled study: The Smiths spoke at the seventy-second annual meeting of the American Gynecological Society held in Hot Springs, Virginia, May 16–18, 1949. When their presentation appeared in print, it included the lengthy discussion that took place after their talk. Olive Watkins Smith and George Van S. Smith, "The Influence of Diethylstilbestrol on the Progress and Outcome of Pregnancy as Based on a Comparison of Treated with Untreated Primigravidas," *American Journal of Obstetrics and Gynecology* 58 (November 1949): 994–1009.

121 Dieckmann four years later: The seventy-sixth annual meeting of the American Gynecology Society took place in Lake Placid, New York from June 15–17, 1953. Dieckmann's presentation and the discussion that followed appear in William J. Dieckmann, M. E. Davis, L. M. Rynkiewicz, and R. E. Pottinger, "Does the Administration of Diethylstilbestrol during Pregnancy Have a Therapeutic Value," *American Journal of Obstetrics and Gynecology* 66 (November 1953): 1062–81. A reanalysis of the Dieckmann study done after the dangers of DES surfaced showed that the treated women actually had nearly twice as many miscarriages as the untreated women. See Yvonne Brackbill and Heinz W. Berendes, "Dangers of Diethylstilboestrol: Review of a 1953 Paper," *Lancet* 2 (September 2, 1978): 520.

122 Important differences in trial design: While the 1949 study reported by the

Smiths restricted participants to first-time pregnant women who had no other health problems, the Dieckmann study included those who had such "complications" as diabetes and hypertension. The Dieckmann group also studied DES in women who previously had had miscarriages, as well as those who had other children. The Dieckmann study had another serious weakness that today would receive much scrutiny: it enrolled 2,162 patients, but could analyze the results from only 1,646. This high "dropout" rate weakens the ultimate findings because researchers do not know what they do not have: It could be that the reason women did not complete the study as planned was connected to DES's success or failure.

122   again stunned the medical community: Arthur L. Herbst, Robert J. Kurman, and Robert E. Scully, "Vaginal and Cervical Abnormalities after Exposure to Stilbestrol in Utero," *Obstetrics & Gynecology* 40 (September 1972): 287–98.

123   Kaufman presented their findings: The conference, the eighty-seventh annual meeting of the Association of Obstetricians and Gynecologists, took place in Hot Springs, Virginia, September 9–11, 1976. The presentation and the subsequent discussion appeared in Raymond H. Kaufman, Gary L. Binder, Paul Milton Gray, Jr., and Ervin Adam, "Upper Genital Tract Changes with Exposure in Utero to Diethylstilbestrol," *American Journal of Obstetrics and Gynecology* 128 (May 1, 1977): 51–59.

125   "long and convoluted saga": Roy M. Pitkin, "Classic Article: Vaginal and Cervical Abnormailties after Exposure to Stilbestrol in Utero," *Obstetrics & Gynecology* 102 (August 2003): 222.

126   676 DES daughters: Kaufman first reported this finding at the second annual meeting of the American Gynecological and Obstetrical Society, held in Phoenix, Arizona, on September 7–10, 1983. The presentation and subsequent discussion appeared in Raymond H. Kaufman, Kenneth Noller, Ervin Adam, et al., "Upper Genital Tract Abnormalities and Pregnancy Outcome in Diethylstilbestrol-exposed Progeny," *American Journal of Obstetrics and Gynecology* 148 (April 1, 1984): 973–84.

126   This remarkable study: Raymond H. Kaufman, Ervin Adam, Elizabeth E. Hatch, et al., "Continued Follow-Up of Pregnancy Outcomes in Diethylstilbestrol-exposed Offspring," *Obstetrics & Gynecology* 96 (October 2000): 483–89. The infertility data appear in a different publication cowritten by many of the same authors. See Julie R. Palmer, Elizabeth E. Hatch, R. Sowmya Rao, et al., "Infertility among Women Exposed Prenatally to Diethylstilbestrol," *American Journal of Epidemiology* 154 (2001): 316–21. The specific analysis of reproductive outcome in women with T-shaped uteri appeared in the 1984 paper that looked at 676 DES daughters, 327 of whom had become pregnant. One obvious limitation: Because the women had an average age of thirty years old, they had

several more reproductive years during which they might have become pregnant and carried to term.

126   successful surgical repair of T-shaped uteri: Olivier Garbin, Jeanine Ohl, Karima Bettahar-Lebugle, and Pierre Dellenbach, "Hysteroscopic Metroplasty in Diethylstilboestrol-exposed and Hypoplastic Uterus: A Report on 24 Cases," *Human Reproduction* 13 (1998): 2751–55.

127   whether DES harmed males: In 2003, the U.S. Centers for Disease Control and Prevention launched a DES Web site, www.cdc.gov/des, which thoroughly reviews the different known and suspected harmful effects of the drug.

127   a 2003 meta-analysis: Anthony A. Bamigboye and J. Morris, "Oestrogen Supplementation, Mainly Diethylstilbestrol, for Preventing Miscarriages and Other Adverse Pregnancy Outcomes," Cochrane Library 4 (2003).

128   the Food and Drug Administration failed: Several studies done shortly after the synthesis of DES showed that it caused cancer in animal experiments. See Dolores Ibarreta and Shanna H. Swan, "The DES Story: Long-term Consequences of Prenatal Exposure," Chapter 8 in *Late Lessons from Early Warnings: The Precautionary Principle 1896 2000*, Environmental issue report No. 22, European Environment Agency, Luxembourg: Office for Official Publications of the European Communities, 2001. Indeed, DES's unintended actions date back to its original synthesis. In *DES: The Bitter Pill* (p. 41), Robert Meyers interviewed a collaborator of Charles Dodds's, who noted that when he first synthesized the drug, powder flew around the lab and several of the workmen developed such large breasts that they "had problems putting their braces [suspenders] on."

129   in their 1952 report of DES's failure: David Robinson and Landrum Shettles, "The Use of Diethylstilbestrol in Threatened Abortion," *American Journal of Obstetrics and Gynecology* 63 (1952): 1330–33. Shettles later won much attention for his own string of controversies. He cowrote with David Rorick a widely read book, *How to Choose the Sex of Your Baby: The Method Best Supported by Scientific Evidence*, first published in 1970 and still in print (Doubleday, 1997). In a July 25, 1999, *New York Times Magazine* article, "Getting the Girl," the writer Lisa Belkin noted that the medical establishment dismissed the Shettles method and other sex-selection theories as "so much hocus-pocus." Shettles, an in vitro fertilization pioneer, in 1978 also found himself embroiled in a court case over the destruction of an embryo he helped a couple create five years earlier. See Judith Cummings, "Test-Tube Case Hears Evidence On Dr. Shettles," *New York Times*, p. B2. In 1994, when London's *Daily Mail* broke the infamous story (mentioned in the preceding chapter) about Malcolm Pearce's fraudulent experiment that supposedly showed how to rescue an ectopic pregnancy, Shettles came to Pearce's defense, telling the paper, "I have no doubt Mr. Pearce did

succeed." See Jenny Hope and Greg Hadfield, "Baby Doctors in Hoax Probe; Cloud Over Operation that Gave Hope to Thousands of Women," *Daily Mail*, November 17, 1994, p. 1.

8: ANATOMICALLY INCORRECT

130 "something uncomfortable coming down below": Lesley Regan recounts this story in her book, *Miscarriage: What Every Woman Needs to Know*, London: Orion Books, 2001, p. 42. I also discussed this case with her. The quotations come from both my interviews and her book.

130 a ridiculous range of conclusions: Antonio Pellicer, "Shall We Operate on Müllerian Defects? An Introduction to the Debate," *Human Reproduction* 12 (1997): 1371–72.

131 An excellent overview: Grigoris F. Grimbizis, Michel Camus, Basil C. Tarlatzis, et al., "Clinical Implications of Uterine Malformations and Hysteroscopic Treatment Results," *Human Reproduction Update* 7 (2001): 161–74.

131 the developmental process that transforms: Paul C. Lin, Kunwar P. Bhatnagar, G. Stephen Nettleton, et al., "Female Genital Anomalies Affecting Reproduction," *Fertility and Sterility* 78 (November 2002): 899–915. For superb illustrations of each uterine anomaly, see Ibrahim Syed, "Uterus, Müllerian Duct Anomalies": http://www.emedicine.com/radio/topic738.htm.

132 astonishing success rates: This remarkable report comes from the clinician who invented the most commonly used surgical technique to repair anomalous uteri. E. O. Strassmann, "Fertility and Unification of a Double Uterus," *Fertility and Sterility* 17 (1966): 165–76.

132 As often occurs in the surgical field: Todd R. Jenkins, "It's Time to Challenge Surgical Dogma with Evidence-based Data," *American Journal of Obstetrics and Gynecology* 189 (August 2003): 423–27.

132 its own eponymous journal: The Web site for Oxford's Centre for Evidence-Based Medicine has a thorough overview of the subject: http://www.cebm.net.

132 centers at leading universities: A dozen evidence-based centers now exist in the United Kingdom, including one at Oxford University. The U.S. Agency for Healthcare Research and Quality as of June 2002 funded thirteen evidence-based centers at universities and think tanks in the United States and Canada.

134 bed rest, another unproven intervention: One 1994 review of the literature found no evidence that bed rest prevents first-trimester miscarriages, and saw little benefit except in cases of preeclampsia. The researchers concluded that unnecessary hospitalizations and lost wages might amount to more than $1 billion per year. Robert L. Goldenberg, Suzanne P. Cliver, Janet Bronstein, et al., "Bed Rest in Pregnancy," *Obstetrics & Gynecology* 84 (July 1994): 131–36. See

also Caroline Crowther, "Bed Rest for Women with Pregnancy Problems: Evidence for Efficacy Is Lacking," *Birth* 22 (1995): 13–14. Bed rest presents physical and emotional risks, too. See Maureen Heaman and Annette Gupton, "Perceptions of Bed Rest by Women with High-Risk Pregnancies: A Comparison Between Home and Hospital," *Birth* 25 (1998): 252–58.

137   More than four decades: V. N. Shirodkar first described transvaginal cerclage at a 1951 convention of the French Gynecological Association. See Sietske M. Althuisius, Gustaaf A. Dekker, and Herman P. Van Geijn, "Cervical Incompetence: A Reappraisal of an Obstetric Controversy," *Obstetrical and Gynecological Survey* 57 (2002): 377–87.

137   "crude, archaic procedure": James H. Harger, "Poor Design in Cerclage Studies," *American Journal of Obstetrics and Gynecology* 186 (March 2002): 594–95.

137   That same year: James H. Harger, "Cerclage and Cervical Insufficiency: An Evidence-Based Analysis," *Obstetrics & Gynecology* 100 (December 2002): 1313–27.

138   factors that cause the cervix to weaken: In one study involving 636 women who attended a recurrent miscarriage clinic, 25 percent had had a second-trimester loss. Of these women, one-third tested positive for antiphospholipid syndrome. Andrew J. Drakeley, Siobhan Quenby, and Roy G. Farquharson, "Mid-trimester Loss—Appraisal of a Screening Program," *Human Reproduction* 13 (1998): 1975–80. Researchers convincingly linked DES to cervical incompetence in several studies, including Jack Ludmir, Mark B. Landon, Steven G. Gabbe, et al., "Management of the Diethylstilbestrol-exposed Patient: Prospective Study," *American Journal of Obstetrics and Gynecology* 157 (1987): 665–69. For an overview of other possible causes, see Errol R. Norwitz, "Emergency Cerclage: What Do the Data Really Show?" *Contemporary OB/GYN* 10 (October 1, 2002): 48–66.

138   transvaginal ultrasound to measure their cervixes: Jay D. Iams, Robert L. Goldenberg, Paul J. Meis, et al., "The Length of the Cervix and the Risk of Spontaneous Premature Delivery," *New England Journal of Medicine* 334 (February 29, 1996): 567–72.

139   One study of 194 women: The two studies appeared back to back. The smaller one was done by R. W. Rush, S. Isaacs, K. McPherson, et al., "A Randomized Controlled Trial of Cervical Cerclage in Women at High Risk of Spontaneous Preterm Delivery," *British Journal of Obstetrics and Gynaecology* 91 (1984): 724–30. The larger study was done by P. Lazar, S. Gueguen, J. Dreyfus, et al., "Multicentered Controlled Trial of Cervical Cerclage in Women at Moderate Risk of Preterm Delivery," *British Journal of Obstetrics and Gynaecology* 91 (1984): 731–35.

139   A large international study: Medical Research Council/Royal College of Obstetricians and Gynaecologists Working Party on Cervical Cerclage, "Final Report of the Medical Research Council/Royal College of Obstetricians and Gy-

naecologists Multicentre Randomized Trial of Cervical Cerclage," *British Journal of Obstetrics and Gynaecology* 100 (1993): 516–23.

139 At the annual meeting: Orion A. Rust, Robert O. Atlas, Kelly Jo Jones, et al., "A Randomized Trial of Cerclage Versus No Cerclage among Patients with Ultrasonographically Detected Second-Trimester Preterm Dilatation of the Internal Os," *American Journal of Obstetrics and Gynecology* 183 (October 2000): 830–85.

140 Dutch group led by Sietske Althuisius: The Dutch study appeared in the same journal thirteen months later. Sietske M. Althuisius, Gustaaf A. Dekker, Pieter Hummel, et al., "Final Results of the Cervical Incompetence Prevention Randomized Cerclage Trial (CIPRACT): Therapeutic Cerclage with Bed Rest Versus Bed Rest Alone," *American Journal of Obstetrics and Gynecology* 185 (November 2001): 1106–12. The CIPRACT group later published evidence that cerclage and bed rest increased cervical length more than bed rest alone. Sietske M. Althuisius, Gustaaf A. Dekker, Pieter Hummel, et al., "Cervical Incompetence Prevention Randomized Cerclage Trial (CIPRACT): Effect of Therapeutic Cerclage with Bed Rest vs. Bed Rest Only on Cervical Length," *Ultrasound in Obstetrics and Gynecology* 20 (2002): 163–67. For an update on the Pennsylvania study, see Orion A. Rust, Robert O. Atlas, James Reed, et al., "Revisiting the Short Cervix Detected by Transvaginal Ultrasound in the Second Trimester: Why Cerclage Therapy May Not Help," *American Journal of Obstetrics and Gynecology* 185 (November 2001): 1098–1105.

141 A meta-analysis of 2,175 women: Andrew J. Drakeley, Devender Roberts, and Zarko Alfirevic, "Cervical Cerclage for Prevention of Preterm Delivery: Meta-analysis of Randomized Trials," *Obstetrics & Gynecology* 102 (September 2003): 621–27.

142 "It's not grounded": As an example of the type of studies the field lacks, Harger said he would like to see more work similar to that done by Phyllis Leppert of the National Institute of Child Health and Human Development. In rat studies, Leppert and coworkers examined what impact collagen, a fibrous protein, has on the tensile strength of the cervix. See Phyllis Leppert, Robert Kokenyesi, C. A. Klemenich, et al., "Further Evidence of a Decorin-Collagen Interaction in the Disruption of Cervical Collagen Fibers during Rat Gestation," *American Journal of Obstetrics and Gynecology* 182 (2000): 805–11.

143 in at least 20 percent of women: Postmortem studies have shown a range of 20 percent to 50 percent, according to Edmund R. Novak and J. Donald Woodruff, "Myoma and Other Benign Tumors of the Uterus," *Gynecologic and Obstetric Pathology*, 8th Edition, Philadelphia: W. B. Saunders, 1979, pp. 260–78. A study of one hundred uteri analyzed after hysterectomy found fibroids in 77 percent of the samples. See Stewart F. Cramer and A. Patel, "The Frequency of Uterine Leiomyomas," *American Journal of Clinical Pathology* 94 (October 1990): 435–38.

143   links fibroids to miscarriages: Fibroids technically are called leiomyomata, and the surgery that removes them is a myomectomy. For an overview of fibroids and miscarriage, see Nitu Bajekal and Tin-Chu Li, "Fibroids, Infertility and Pregnancy Wastage," *Human Reproduction Update* 6 (2000): 614–20. A retrospective analysis by researchers at Johns Hopkins University found that women with fibroids diagnosed on ultrasound had an eight-times-higher risk of having a second-trimester miscarriage. Erin Salvador, Jessica Bienstock, Karin J. Blakemore, and Eva Pressman, "Leiomyomata Uteri, Genetic Amniocentesis, and the Risk of Second-Trimester Spontaneous Abortion," *American Journal of Obstetrics and Gynecology* 186 (May 2002): 913–15.

144   more than six hundred articles: Evan R. Myers, Matthew D. Barber, Tara Gustilo-Ashby, et al., "Management of Uterine Leiomyomata: What Do We Really Know?" *Obstetrics & Gynecology* 100 (July 2002): 8–17.

144   all relied on a retrospective analysis: To appreciate the level of confusion a retrospective analysis can create, see Tin-Chu Li, R. Mortimer, and Ian Douglas Cooke, "Myomectomy: A Retrospective Study to Examine Reproductive Performance Before and After Surgery," *Human Reproduction* 14 (1999): 1735–40. This report claims that surgical removal of fibroids "appeared to significantly reduce the occurrence of miscarriage associated with fibroids." But a close analysis shows that this claim rests on data that analyzed a mere eleven patients who had a history of miscarriage. As a control, the study compares these patients to themselves, looking at their collective miscarriage rate before and after the surgery. Their supposed improved success rate might just reflect the high success rate seen in any group of women who miscarry a few times and become pregnant again.

144   Piling several retrospective analyses together: For a superb review of studies that evaluated the links between endometriosis and miscarriage, see Ellen E. Vercammen and Thomas M. D'Hooghe, "Endometriosis and Recurrent Pregnancy Loss," *Seminars in Reproductive Medicine* 18 (2000): 363–68.

144   An article in a 1997 newsletter: Beth Glosten, "Benefits and Pitfalls of Retrospective Studies," "Society for Obstetric Anesthesia and Perinatology Newsletter," Winter 1997.

9: THE SKY ISN'T FALLING

149   In the spring of 1893: "A Model Industrial City," *New York Times*, May 31, 1893, p. 12. Other details about Love's scheme, including the lyrics to his ditty, come from "Love Canal: Public Health Time Bomb," New York State Department of Health, September 1978. See also "Celebration at Niagara Falls: The Hydraulic Canal, It Is Said, Will Be Finished in a Year," *New York Times*, August 1, 1894, p. 4.

150 Anne Hillis composed her own verse: Testimony of Anne Hillis Before the Senate Standing Committee on Conservation and Recreation, Assembly Standing Committee on Environmental Conservation, Senate Subcommittee on Toxic Substances and Chemical Waste, Assembly Environmental Conservation Committee Task Force on Toxic Substances. Niagara Falls International Convention Center, Niagara Falls, New York, May 3, 1979. Available online at the Love Canal Collection, State University of New York at Buffalo, http://ublib.buffalo.edu/libraries/projects/lovecanal. This superb resource contains many of the original documents about Love Canal's history.

151 President Jimmy Carter to propose the legislation: "Carter Proposes $1.6 billion Fund to Fight Chemical Waste Hazards," New York Times, June 14, 1979, p. A1.

151 more than two hundred chemicals: "Love Canal: A Special Report to the Governor and Legislature," New York State Department of Health, April 1981. This thorough overview recounts the toxological and epidemiological investigations in detail.

152 writing into the deed: See Eric Zuesse, "Love Canal: The Truth Seeps Out," Reason, February 1981, pp. 16–33.

152 birds falling from the sky: "Progress Report of the Ecumenical Task Force of the Niagara Frontier, Inc.," March 20, 1979–August 1, 1980, p. xvii. Available online at the Love Canal Collection Web site.

152 His official report: Lawrence R. Moriarty, "Chemical Waste—Love Canal," October 18, 1977. Available online at the Love Canal Collection Web site.

153 issued an emergency declaration: This notice appears as an appendix to "Draft Report: Analysis of a Ground Water Contamination Incident in Niagara Falls, New York," prepared for the U.S. Environmental Protection Agency, Office of Solid Waste, by Fred C. Hart Associates, Inc., July 28, 1978.

153 under the national media's radar: By August 20, the international media had so swarmed the area that the Niagara Gazette did an article about the press invasion. The paper cracked that the town had not had this much publicity since 1960, when a seven-year-old boy was swept over Niagara Falls and survived. See Mark Francis, "Reporters Flock to Canal Crisis," Niagara Gazette, August 20, 1978. Available online at the Niagara Gazette archive at the Love Canal Connection Web site.

153 "presented a great and imminent peril": Donald G. McNeil, Jr., "Health Chief Calls Waste Site a 'Peril': Asks Pregnant Women and Children to Leave Niagara Falls Sector," New York Times, August 3, 1978, p. B17. This story is the first in the New York Times to cover the Love Canal contamination.

153 Carter approved emergency aid: Donald G. McNeil, Jr., "Carter Approves Emergency Help in Niagara Area," New York Times, August 8, 1978, p. A1.

153 which included testimony from Paigen: Beverly Paigen publicly reported details of her findings to the U.S. House Subcommittee on Oversight and Investigations, March 21, 1979. Her testimony and Anne Hillis's are available online at the Love Canal Connection Web site.

154 Hillis, who had lost one baby: Hillis mentioned losing a child at the hearing, but did not go into details. She did describe the loss in detail to reporters, however. Michael H. Brown, the reporter for the *Niagara Gazette* who led the paper's coverage of Love Canal, made mention of Hillis's miscarriage in "Love Canal and the Poisoning of America," *The Atlantic Monthly*, December 1979, pp. 33–47. See also Dudley Clendinen, "Love Canal: A Boyhood Is Poisoned," *New York Times*, June 19, 1980, p. B1.

154 the outcomes in nearly seven thousand pregnancies: Dorothy Warburton and F. Clarke Fraser, "Spontaneous Abortion Risks in Man: Data from Reproductive Histories Collected in a Medical Genetics Unit," *Human Genetics* 16 (March 1964): 1–25.

156 Beverly Paigen's analysis: Lois M. Gibbs, the head of the Love Canal Homeowners Association, testified on March 21, 1979, to the House Subcommittee on Oversight and Investigation about the first results from Paigen's study. She noted that the health department on October 25, 1978, announced that "there is no evidence to date indicating that miscarriage rates among women in the reproductive age group who live [further away from the canal] exceeded expected levels." According to Gibbs, her citizens group gave the state health department an analysis on December 20, 1978, which showed a "better than two-fold increase" in miscarriages in the homes that had yet to be evacuated.

156 The findings hardly made a compelling case: Nicholas J. Vianna, Adele K. Polan, Ronald Regal, et al., "Adverse Pregnancy Outcomes in the Love Canal Area," New York State Department of Public Health, Draft, April 1980. Updated, slightly different data appear in "Love Canal: A Special Report to the Governor & Legislature," New York State Department of Health, April 1981. Both are available online at the Love Canal Connection Web site.

157 The findings spurred the New York state health commissioner: Donald G. McNeil, Jr., "100 Love Canal Families Are Urged to Leave Area," *New York Times*, February 10, 1979, p. 21.

157 supposedly had chromosomal abnormalities: Irvin Molotsky, "Damage to Chromosome Found in Love Canal Tests," *New York Times*, May 17, 1980, p. 1.

157 "said the findings completed a cycle of proof": See Josh Barbanel, "Homeowners Are Bitter and Fearful as Results of Study Are Released," *New York Times*, May 18, 1980, p. 1. A few days later, when two EPA officials visited the office of the Love Canal Homeowners Association to discuss the chromosome tests, a crowd of three hundred people gathered outside, and the officials were told

they could not leave. "We are not holding them hostage," insisted Lois Gibbs, head of the association. "We're protecting them because the crowd outside will tear them apart." After five hours, agents from the Federal Bureau of Investigation ordered the residents to let the environmental officials leave. See Josh Barbanel, "Homeowners at Love Canal Hold 2 Officials Until F.B.I. Intervenes," *New York Times*, May 20, 1980, p. 1.

157   caused these maladies: For a more detailed, critical account of the chromosome analysis, see Gina Bari Kolata, "Love Canal: False Alarm Caused by Botched Study," *Science* 208 (June 13, 1980): 1239–42. Also see Richard Severo, Richard Meislin, Robert Reinhold, et al., "A Tangle of Science and Politics Lies Behind Study at Love Canal," *New York Times*, May 27, 1980, p. A1.

157   Carter declared another federal emergency: Irvin Molotsky, "President Orders Emergency Help for Love Canal," *New York Times*, May 22, 1980, p. 1.

157   That June, New York Governor Hugh Carey: "Report of the Governor's Panel to Review Scientific Studies and the Development of Public Policy on Problems Resulting from Hazardous Wastes," October 8, 1980, available online at the Love Canal Collection Web site. Following an article in *Science* about the report, Beverly Paigen wrote a letter to the editor in her own defense, explaining that her study "was never intended as a definitive epidemiological survey," yet also emphasizing that her findings about adverse pregnancy outcomes had been "replicated by the New York State Department of Health." See Beverly Paigen, Letters, *Science* 211 (January 2, 1981): 6 and 8.

158   a stack of scientific papers: For a paper that cites several of these reports, see Beverly Paigen, Lynn R. Goldman, Mary M. Magnat, et al., "Growth of Children Living Near the Hazardous Waste Site, Love Canal," *Human Biology* 59 (June 1987): 489–508.

159   the health of the voles: M. H. Rowley, J. J. Christian, D. K. Basu, et al., "Use of Small Mammals (Voles) to Assess a Hazardous Waste Site at Love Canal, Niagara Falls, New York," *Archives of Environmental Contamination and Toxicology* 12 (1983): 383–97.

159   before responding to a bomb threat: Beverly Paigen, "Controversy at Love Canal," *Hastings Center Report* 12 (June 1982): 29–37.

160   become a made-for-television movie: *Lois Gibbs and the Love Canal*, CBS, 1982.

161   in one smoking study: Jennie Kline, Bruce Levin, Ann Kinney, et al., "Cigarette Smoking and Spontaneous Abortion of Known Karyotype: Precise Data but Uncertain Inferences," *American Journal of Epidemiology* 141 (1995): 417–27.

162   Would that more of the journalists: Jennifer R. Gardella and Joseph A. Hill III, "Environmental Toxins Associated with Recurrent Pregnancy Loss," *Seminars in Reproductive Medicine* 18 (2000): 407–24.

163   a famous 1988 study: Marilyn K. Goldhaber, Michael R. Polen, and Robert A.

Hiatt, "The Risk of Miscarriage and Birth Defects among Women Who Use Visual Display Terminals during Pregnancy," *American Journal of Industrial Medicine* 13 (1988): 695–706. The study made a big splash in the media. See Lawrence K. Altman, "Pregnant Women's Use of VDTs Is Scrutinized," *New York Times*, June 5, 1988, section 1, p. 22.

164   more than 20,000 pregnant Danish women: Ulrik Kesmodel, Kirsten Wisborg, Sjurdur Frodi Olsen, et al., "Moderate Alcohol Intake in Pregnancy and the Risk of Spontaneous Abortion," *Alcohol and Alcoholism* 37 (2002): 87–92.

164   a striking increase in miscarriage related to alcohol use: Jennie Kline, P. Shrout, Zeta Stein, et al., "Drinking during Pregnancy and Spontaneous Abortion," *Lancet* 2 (July 26, 1980): 176–80.

165   researchers from the California Department of Health Services: Shanna Swan, Kirsten Waller, Barbara Hopkins, et al., "A Prospective Study of Spontaneous Abortion: Relation to Amount and Source of Drinking Water Consumed in Early Pregnancy," *Epidemiology* 9 (March 1998): 126–33.

165   Page-one articles appeared in the *Los Angeles Times*: Jim Newton and Julie Marquis, "Tap Water Linked to Miscarriages," *Los Angeles Times*, February 10, 1998, p. 1. Jim Newton and Thomas Maugh II, "Water Officials Suggest Prudence, Not Panic," *Los Angeles Times*, February 11, 1998. Julia Scheeres and Abigail Goldman, "New Worry for Pregnant Women," *Los Angeles Times*, February 11, 1998, p. 1. Also see the follow-up story, Julie Marquis, "Caution Urged in Reacting to Tap Water Scare," *Los Angeles Times*, February 19, 1998.

166   cause no harm to embryos or fetuses: Joe Leigh Simpson, a leading miscarriage researcher at Baylor College of Medicine in Houston, looked with his colleagues at the role of infection in two, large prospective studies of miscarriage. They found no impact, leading them to conclude that "extant data do not provide evidence that clinically evident infections play major roles in first-trimester pregnancy losses." See Joe Leigh Simpson, James L. Mills, H. Kim, et al., "Infectious Processes: An Infrequent Cause of First-Trimester Spontaneous Abortions," *Human Reproduction* 11 (March 1996): 668–72. Also see Joe Leigh Simpson, Ronald H. Gray, John T. Queenan, et al., "Further Evidence That Infection Is an Infrequent Cause of First-Trimester Spontaneous Abortion," *Human Reproduction* 11 (September 1996): 2058–60.

166   a few pathogens may account: To make these references easier to read, I have divided them by disease, indicated in bold type. A large U.S. epidemic of **rubella** in 1964 and 1965 "left behind a wake of abnormal infants and terminated pregnancies," wrote Stanley Plotkin, a leading expert on rubella vaccines. See Stanley A. Plotkin and Edward A. Mortimer, *Vaccines*, Philadelphia: W. B. Saunders Company, 1998, p. 235. For a detailed study of that epidemic, see A.W. Karchmer, G. Case, et al., "Epidemiology of Rubella," *American Journal of*

Diseases of Children 118 (1969): 107–12. I contacted Plotkin about rubella and miscarriage, and he also recommended reading S. J. Sallomi, "Rubella in Pregnancy. A Review of Prospective Studies from the Literature," *Obstetrics & Gynecology* 27 (February 1966): 252–56. For recent **syphilis** studies, see Deborah Watson-Jones, John Changalucha, Balthazar Gumodoka, et al., "Syphilis in Pregnancy in Tanzania. I. Impact of Maternal Syphilis on Outcome of Pregnancy," *Journal of Infectious Diseases* 186 (2002): 940–47. For an authoritative **genital herpes** study, see Andre Nahmias, William E. Josey, Zuher M. Naib, et al., "Perinatal Risk Associated with Maternal Genital Herpes Simplex Virus Infection," *American Journal of Obstetrics and Gynecology* 110 (July 15, 1971): 825–37. Also see M. D. Libman, A. Dascal, M. S. Kramer, et al., "Strategies for the Prevention of Neonatal Infection with Herpes Simplex Virus: A Decision Analysis," *Review of Infectious Diseases* 13 (1991): 1093–1104. For **mumps,** see M. Siegel, "Congenital Malformations Following Chickenpox, Measles, Mumps, and Hepatitis," *Journal of the American Medical Association* 226 (December 24, 1973): 1521–24. **Toxoplasmosis** causes miscarriage in sheep and other domesticated animals, but the human data remain unclear. See Patrick Hohlfeld, Fernand Daffos, Jean-Marc Costa, et al., "Prenatal Diagnosis of Congenital Toxoplasmosis with a Polymerase-Chain-Reaction Test on Amniotic Fluid," *New England Journal of Medicine* 331 (September 15, 1994): 695–99. The impact of **malaria** on miscarriage remains especially tricky to ferret out because the disease primarily occurs in countries that do not offer pregnant women much prenatal care, meaning that no one tracks miscarriages. It seems that different strains of the parasite that causes malaria appear to affect pregnant women differently, with some possibly triggering miscarriages while others do not. See Francis Nosten, R. McGready, J. A. Simpson, et al., "Effects of *Plasmodium vivax* Malaria in Pregnancy," *Lancet* 354 (August 14, 1999): 546–49. For *Plasmodium falciparum,* see Robert D. Newman, Monica E. Parise, Laurence Slutsker, et al., *Tropical Medicine & International Health* 8 (June 2003): 488–506. The two largest **HIV/AIDS** studies — one retrospective, one prospective — had conflicting results about whether the infection increased miscarriage rates. See Carlo D'Ubaldo, Patrizio Pezzotti, Giovanni Rezza, et al., "Association Between HIV-1 Infection and Miscarriage: A Retrospective Study," *AIDS* 12 (1998): 1087–93. Also see Birgit H. B. van Benthem, Isabelle de Vincenzi, Marie-Christine Delmas, et al., "Pregnancies Before and After HIV Diagnosis in a European Cohort of HIV-Infected Women," *AIDS* 14 (2000): 2171–78. William Shearer's group at Baylor also has proposed an interesting miscarriage mechanism that involves HIV's impact on the thymus and the immune system. William Shearer, C. Langston, D. E. Lewis, et al., "Early Spontaneous Abortions and Fetal Thymic Abnormalities in Maternal-to-Fetal HIV Infection," *Acta Paediatrics* 421 Supplement (1997): 60–64.

166 They can lead to stillbirths, too: Stillbirth, usually defined as a fetal death after at least twenty weeks gestation, overlaps with miscarriage, but the two topics ultimately present unique causes and interventions, and I consistently have attempted to separate them. For a deep-dish review of the relationship between infections and stillbirth, see Robert L. Goldenberg and Cortney Thompson, "The Infectious Origins of Stillbirth," *American Journal of Obstetrics and Gynecology* 189 (September 2003): 861–73.

166 an exotic-sounding list of bugs: Again, I have separated by disease, indicated in bold type. *Listeria monocytogenes* unquestionably causes miscarriages in farm animals, but the human data remain decidedly more spotty. See Helayne M. Silver, "Listeriosis During Pregnancy," *Obstetrical & Gynecological Survey* 53 (December 1998): 737–40. For a **Parvovirus B19** review, see Roni Levy, Ariel Weissman, Gary Blomberg, et al., "Infection by Parvovirus B 19 During Pregnancy," *Obstetrical and Gynecological Survey* 52 (April 1997): 254–59. Parvovirus B19 seems particularly linked to second trimester miscarriages. See Public Health Laboratory Service Working Party of Fifth Disease, "Prospective Study of Human Parvovirus (B19) Infection in Pregnancy," *British Medical Journal* 300 (May 5, 1990): 1166–70. Evidence remains sketchy for a clear link between **cytomegalovirus** and miscarriage, in part because the virus has become so ubiquitous. See L. C. Spano, P. R. M. Vargasa, F. S. Ribeirob, et al., "Cytomegalovirus in Human Abortion in Espírito Santo, Brazil," *Journal of Clinical Virology* 25 Supplement 2 (August 2002): 173–78. *Ureaplasma urealyticum* similarly is common and thus difficult to convict definitively as a cause of miscarriage. See "Relationship of Bacterial Vaginosis and Mycoplasmas to the Risk of Spontaneous Abortion," *American Journal of Obstetrics and Gynecology* 183 (August 2000): 431–37. For an overview of studies that treated *Gardnerella vaginalis* and *Mycoplasma hominis,* see S. G. Ralph, A. J. Rutherford, and J. D. Wilson, "Influence of Bacterial Vaginosis on Conception and Miscarriage in the First Trimester," *British Medical Journal* 319 (1999): 220–23.

171 an investigation of a miscarriage cluster: "Spontaneous Abortions Possibly Related to Ingestion of Nitrate-Contaminated Well Water—LaGrange County, Indiana, 1991–1994," *Morbidity and Mortality Weekly Report* 45 (July 5, 1996): 569–72.

173 thrust Hunt's lab into the middle of the controversial field: Patricia A. Hunt, Kara E. Koehler, Martha Susiarjo, et al., "Bisphenol A Exposure Causes Meiotic Aneuploidy in the Female Mouse," *Current Biology* 13 (April 1, 2003): 546–53. See also Kara E. Koehler, S. Thomas, Bruce Lamb, et al., "When Disaster Strikes: Rethinking Caging Materials," *Lab Animal* 32 (April 2003): 32–35.

173 argued that low levels of certain synthetic chemicals: For a thorough overview, see Wade V. Welshons, Kristina A. Thayer, Barbara M. Judy, et al., "Large Ef-

fects from Small Exposures. I. Mechanisms for Endocrine-Disrupting Chemicals with Estrogenic Activity," *Environmental Health Perspectives* 111 (June 2003): 994–1006.

10: EXPERT CARE

175   one of the most peculiar miscarriage studies: Babill Stray-Pedersen and Sverre Stray-Pedersen, "Etiologic Factors and Subsequent Reproductive Performance in 195 Couples with a Prior History of Habitual Abortion," *American Journal of Obstetrics and Gynecology* 148 (1984): 140–46.

176   more evidence that TLC had spectacular powers: Hilary S. Liddell, Neil Pattison, and Angi Zanderigo, "Recurrent Miscarriage — Outcome after Supportive Care in Early Pregnancy," *Australian and New Zealand Journal of Obstetrics and Gynaecology* 31 (1991): 320–22.

180   more than two-thirds of pregnant women: Although researchers typically define recurrent miscarriage as three or more, some use two as the cutoff. Researchers at Liverpool Women's Hospital in 1999 reported that of 226 women they followed who had no identified cause for their previous miscarriages (one-fourth had only two), 75 percent carried to term after receiving no treatment other than tender-loving care. S. A. Brigham, C. Conlon, and R. G. Farquharson, "A Longitudinal Study of Pregnancy Outcome Following Idiopathic Recurrent Miscarriage," *Human Reproduction* 14 (1999): 2868–71. The St. Mary's Hospital Recurrent Miscarriage Clinic found that 69 percent of 201 pregnant women with at least three previous miscarriages had a success without medical intervention. Katy Clifford, Raj Rai, and Lesley Regan, "Future Pregnancy Outcome in Unexplained Recurrent First-Trimester Miscarriage," *Human Reproduction* 12 (February 1997): 387–89. When lumping together treated and untreated patients in these tender-loving-care studies, the success rates were 66 percent in the Norwegian study and 77 percent in the New Zealand one.

189   When apprised of the situation: The Wellcome Library for the History and Understanding of Medicine has a substantial file (GC/150) on Aleck William Bourne. In particular, see: *Rex v. Bourne*, Statement of Dr. A. W. Bourne; a paper by Bourne's daughter, Joan Ostry; and *Rex v. Bourne* and the Medicalisation of Abortion by Barbara Brookes and Paul Roth.

191   backed the tender-loving-care thesis: See Katy Clifford et al., "Future Pregnancy Outcome."

192   multiples frequently "vanish" early in pregnancy: See Helain J. Landy and L. G. Keith, "The Vanishing Twin: A Review," *Human Reproduction Update* 4 (1998): 177–83.

199   new evidence from a prospective study: I discuss thromboelastography and
       this specific study in chapter 5.

11: MIRACLE BABIES

201   one of at least two she suffered: When she was eighteen, Frida Kahlo was rid-
       ing a bus in Mexico City that collided with a streetcar. She broke many bones,
       including her pelvis, and a handrail speared her abdomen, exiting through her
       vagina. The horrible traffic accident would cause her physical problems for the
       rest of her life and, as biographers have speculated, may well have had a link
       to her miscarriages. See Hayden Herrera, *Frida: A Biography of Frida Kahlo* (New
       York: Harper and Row, 1983).

205   As Wilton and her colleagues reported: Leeanda Wilton, Robert Williamson,
       John McBain, et al., "Birth of a Healthy Infant after Preimplantation Confir-
       mation of Euploidy by Comparative Genomic Hybridization," *New England Jour-
       nal of Medicine* 345 (November 22, 2001): 1537–41. In the same issue, see also
       the thoughtful editorial (pp. 1569–71) by Sherman Elias.

205   a study in her clinic of 285 patients: Mary D. Stephenson, Khalid A. Awartani,
       and Wendy P. Robinson, "Cytogenetic Analysis of Miscarriages from Couples
       with Recurrent Miscarriage: A Case-Control Study," *Human Reproduction* 17
       (February 2002): 446–51. I also discuss this study in chapter 3.

206   two sobering studies: For Wilton's group, see Lucille Voullaire, Howard Slater,
       Robert Williamson, et al., "Chromosome Analysis of Blastomeres from Human
       Embryos by Using Comparative Genomic Hybridization," *Human Genetics* 106
       (2000): 210–17. Also see Dagan Wells and Joy D. A. Delhanty, "Comprehensive
       Chromosomal Analysis of Human Preimplantation Embryos Using Whole
       Genome Amplification and Single Cell Comparative Genomic Hybridization,"
       Molecular Human Reproduction 6 (2000): 1055–62.

206   can trigger mosaicism: Santiago Munné, M. Christina Magli, Alexis Adler, et
       al., "Treatment-related Chromosome Abnormalities in Human Embryos,"
       Human Reproduction 12 (1997): 780–84.

206   only about four hundred pregnancies had occurred worldwide: "Tenth An-
       niversary of Preimplantation Genetic Diagnosis," *Journal of Assisted Reproduction
       and Genetics* 18 (2001): 64–70.

207   Roughly seven out of ten transferred embryos miscarry: In collaboration with
       the Society for Assisted Reproductive Technology and the American Society for
       Reproductive Medicine, the U.S. Centers for Disease Control and Prevention
       monitors success rates of assisted reproduction technologies, and most fer-
       tility clinics in the country supply data. In 2001, U.S. clinics made and trans-
       ferred some 65,000 fresh embryos from women's own eggs. Of these, fewer

than 22,000 resulted in a live birth, a failure rate of 69 percent. See "2001 Assisted Reproductive Technology Success Rates," U.S. Centers for Disease Control and Prevention, U.S. Department of Health and Human Services, December 2003.

207 Given better tools: Comparative genomic hybridization or FISH may soon become speeded up through microarray technology, which puts matrixes of DNA onto silicon chips. See Heinz-Ulli G. Weier, Santiago Munné, Robert A. Lersch, et al., "Towards a Full Karyotype Screening of Interphase Cells: 'FISH and Chip' Technology," *Molecular and Cellular Endocrinology* 183 (2001): S41–45. Also see Dagan Wells and Brynn Levy, "Cytogenetics in Reproductive Medicine: The Contribution of Comparative Genomic Hybridization (CGH)," *BioEssays* 25 (2003): 289–300.

GLOSSARY

Abortion: The early expulsion of an embryo or fetus. The common use of the word refers to what doctors call an "induced" abortion. A "spontaneous" abortion refers to a miscarriage. A "threatened" abortion refers to spotting or cramping during pregnancy, typically before the twentieth week of gestation.

Abortus: The miscarried embryo or fetus. See also **products of conception**

Amniocentesis: Also called an "amnio," a procedure that places a needle in the amniotic sac and removes fluid for genetic testing

Aneuploidy: Too few or too many chromosomes

Antibody: Y-shaped protein that latches onto an antigen, blocking its actions

Antigen: A molecule that triggers an immune response

Antiphospholipid syndrome: An autoimmune reaction in which cardiolipin and lupus anticoagulant antibodies are elevated and may cause clots, heart disease, joint pain, and other symptoms

Blastocyst: The ball of cells that separates into what will become the placenta and the embryo

Blastomere: One cell of the early, multicelled embyro

Blighted ovum: A fertilized egg that has no embryo visible on an ultrasound

Cerclage: An operation to close the cervix and prevent preterm delivery, typically done with a suture or surgical tape

Cervix: The opening to the uterus

Cesarean section (C-section): A surgical incision in the abdomen to remove a baby

Chorionic villi sampling (CVS): A procedure that places a needle through the abdomen or a catheter through the cervix to remove placental tissue for genetic testing

Chromosomes: Strands of DNA in the nucleus of cells that hold genetic information

Clomid: Chemically known as clomiphene citrate, this drug stimulates ovulation by blocking the effects of estrogen

Comparative genomic hybridization (CGH): A technique used for both karyotyping miscarriages and biopsied cells during preimplantation genetic diagnosis

Conceptus: The catchall term used to describe the product of conception at every stage of development, all the way up to birth

Corpus luteum: The progesterone-secreting tissue formed by a follicle after it releases an egg

Dilation and curettage (D and C): The opening of the cervix and scraping of the uterus to remove an embryo or fetus

Embryo: The conceptus during the first eight weeks, before it develops a recognizable form

Endometrium: The lining of the uterus

Endometriosis: A condition in which the endometrial tissue grows outside the uterus

Environmental Protection Agency (EPA): The branch of the U.S. government that sets and enforces environmental regulations

Euploidy: A normal complement of forty-six chromosomes

Fallopian tubes: The two canals through which an egg travels on its journey from ovary to uterus

Fetus: The conceptus from the eighth week until birth

Fibroid: A benign tumor (also called a leiomyoma) that can grow in the uterus

Follicle: The husk of cells that surround a maturing egg until its release at ovulation

Food and Drug Administration (FDA): The U.S. agency that regulates the sale of medicine and medical devices

Gestational age: The age of the conceptus from the time of the last menstrual period

Hormone: A biochemical produced in one tissue or organ which travels through the bloodstream and affects a different organ

Human chorionic gonadotropin (hCG): The hormone secreted by the placenta at implantation. Its presence (or absence) is the key to home pregnancy tests.

Hysterosalpingogram: An X-ray of the uterus and fallopian tubes in which an injected dye may highlight obstructions

Hysteroscopy: A procedure in which a scope is placed through the cervix and into the uterus to look for abnormalities

Incompetent cervix: A cervix that dilates before a baby has come to term. Also called an insufficient cervix

Intravenous immunoglobulin (IVIG): A preparation of antibodies pooled from several people

Induced abortion: See **abortion**

In vitro fertilization (IVF): The laboratory process that combines an egg and sperm to form an embryo

Karyotype: The complete set of chromosomes in an individual

Luteal phase: The portion of the ovulatory cycle that begins at ovulation and ends at menses

Luteal phase defect: Also called luteal phase insufficiency, this disorder prevents the uterine lining from maturing with enough blood and sugar to nourish an implanting embryo.

Lymphocyte: White blood cell

Lymphocyte immune therapy: An unproven treatment that isolates white blood cells from a male and injects them into his female partner to prevent her immune system from attacking a baby because it has his "foreign" proteins

Meiosis: The process of cell division that occurs only in eggs and sperm, halving the complement of chromosomes (in humans, from forty-six to twenty-three)

Mitosis: The process of cell division that leaves a new cell with the same number of chromosomes as the original

Menopause: The point at which a woman stops menstruating

Menstruation: The monthly bleeding, or period, that occurs when the uterine lining sloughs off

Metroplasty: Surgery to correct a uterine abnormality

Miscarriage: The loss of an embryo or fetus before it has reached about twenty weeks

Mosaicism: A condition in which some cells in the same embryo, fetus, child, or adult contain different chromosomes from other cells

Müllerian ducts: Two tubes in the embryo that, in females, partially fuse together to form the upper portion of the vagina, the cervix, the uterus, and the fallopian tubes

Myomectomy: The surgery that removes a fibroid

National Institutes of Health (NIH): Part of the U.S. Department of Health and Human Services, this collection of two dozen institutes and centers serves as the premier funder of biomedical research in the United States

Nuchal fold: The nape of the neck that, if thickened in a fetus, can indicate Down syndrome

Ova: Eggs

Ovaries: The two organs that hold a reserve of eggs, releasing one each month at ovulation

Ovarian reserve: Also called an ovarian pool, the total number of eggs in the ovaries

Ovulation: Release of an egg from an ovary

Polycystic ovary syndrome (PCOS): A hormonal disorder, characterized by enlarged ovaries with the appearance of a "string of pearls" around their surface. Symptoms include infertility, irregular periods, weight problems, and excessive levels of male hormones and the associated hair growth.

Preimplantation genetic diagnosis (PGD): A laboratory test used by in vitro fertilization clinics that assesses the genetic health of embryos before transferring them into a woman's uterus

Products of conception: A miscarried embryo or fetus

Recurrent miscarriage: At least two, but usually three or more, miscarriages

Rh factor: A protein, first discovered in rhesus (Rh) monkeys, that most, but not all, humans have. When a woman without the protein conceives with a man who has it, her body can have a dangerous immune response against the offspring.

Septate uterus: An abnormality in which the **müllerian ducts** do not properly fuse during embryonic development, leaving a wall inside of the uterus

Septum: Muscular tissue that separates a cavity

Spontaneous abortion (SAb): See **abortion**

Stillbirth: Fetal death that occurs after at least twenty weeks of gestation

Teratogen: Any substance that can harm developing embryos and fetuses, such as a virus, drug, or chemical

Threatened miscarriage: Early bleeding or cramping. See **abortion**

Thrombosis: Blocking of a blood vessel by a clot that forms at the site

Ultrasound: A diagnostic machine that uses sound waves to visualize embryos and fetuses, or the resulting picture itself. Wands that send the sounds waves can be placed either on the belly or in the vagina (for a transvaginal ultrasound)

Viability: The point at which a fetus can survive outside of the uterus

Viviparity: The ability of a mother to carry offspring and birth a live baby

Womb: The uterus

Zygote: A fertilized egg

INDEX